COOL

YOGA

TRICKS

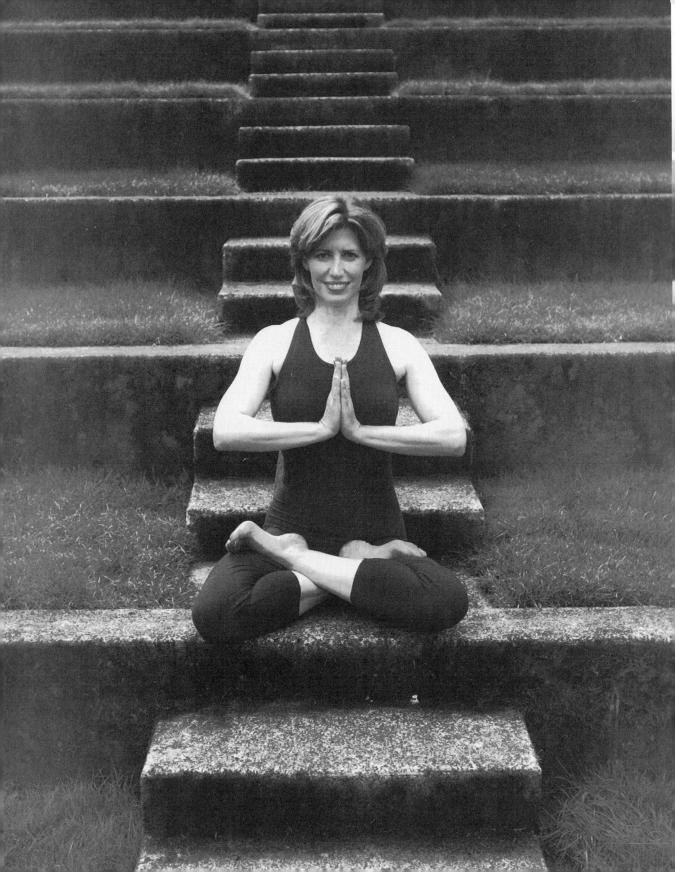

COOL
YOGA
TRICKS

Miriam Austin

BALLANTINE BOOKS / NEW YORK

Author's Note: This book proposes a program of exercise recommendations for the reader to follow. However, you should consult a qualified medical professional (and, if you are pregnant, your ob/gyn) before starting this or any other fitness program. As with any diet or exercise program, if at any time you experience any discomfort, stop immediately and consult your physician.

In gratitude to B.K.S. Iyengar

and to the merciful God who

inspired his genius and who

brought yoga into my life

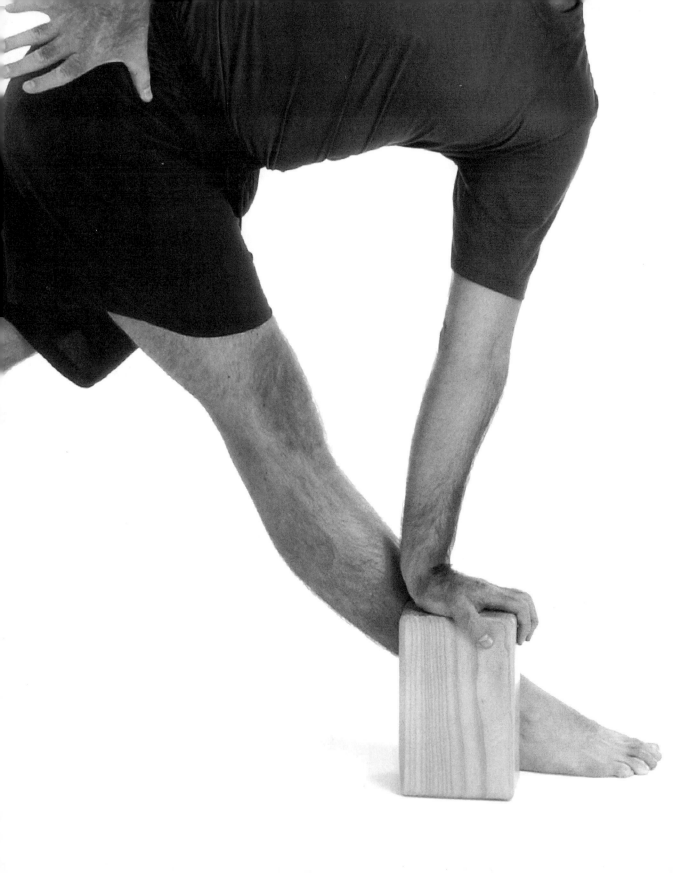

Contents

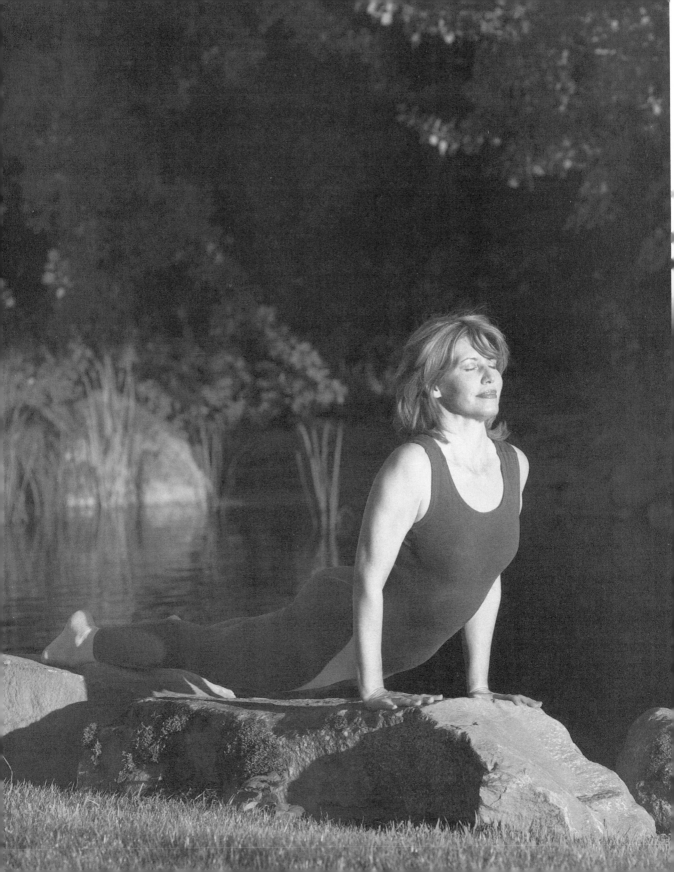

Acknowledgments

This book would have been impossible without the care, concern, and expertise of my most influential teachers, Ramanand Patel and Nancy Stechert. Ramanand and Nancy taught me most of the tricks featured in this book and encouraged me to share these insights with others.

Their teacher, Yogacharya B.K.S. Iyengar, is recognized as the world's leading authority on hatha yoga. Mr. Iyengar developed a method of practicing yoga that includes attention to precision, detailed alignment, and the use of props, which allows students to perform postures they otherwise would not be able to do safely and allows the treatment of many illnesses, injuries, and stress-related conditions. His genius is unsurpassed. Although I say that Mr. Iyengar is my teacher, I have only had the privilege to study with him once.

Over my many years of teaching, my students have become my greatest teachers. Their willingness to trust me and allow me to help them work through their physical, and sometimes emotional, problems is a rare gift. I have asked students to use many of these tricks and their results have left me with a sense of amazement and humility. Many times when students have told me that through yoga they have been cured of a certain injury or illness, I have asked with wonder and surprise, "Do you really think it was the yoga?" When they have assured me that nothing else in their life had changed except the initiation of a yoga practice, I have been awed by and grateful to the mystery that surrounds this ancient discipline.

I am thankful for my literary agent, Michael Broussard, who long before he met me in person had great faith that I would be a successful author.

I could not have been more blessed than to have Maureen O'Neal as my editor at Ballantine Random House. Within a few minutes of our first meeting, she said, "I was born to publish this book." With her great talent, insight, and success with other authors, Maureen was born to do much, much more than this book, but I sincerely appreciate her faith in this project and in me.

I am grateful to the many people at Ballantine Random House who have spent many long hours working on this book. Although I haven't met most of you, I truly appreciate your efforts.

My appreciation for Lubosh Cech, the designer and art director for this book, goes far beyond his extraordinary professional skills. He has become a friend and trusted adviser.

Many thanks to my photographer, Barry Kaplan. Barry has done a magnificent job of capturing the essence and the subtleties of the poses with his discerning eye and camera lens.

The models have helped make this book a visual treat. You are all an inspiration and I thank all of you for your enthusiasm.

Special thanks to Wally Chapman, our makeup artist, who helped us all look our best.

While writing this book, I neglected my husband, family, and friends. Thank you for enduring my absence so patiently.

I am eternally grateful that I have been given the opportunity to write this book. Thanks to everyone who made that possible— particularly you, the reader.

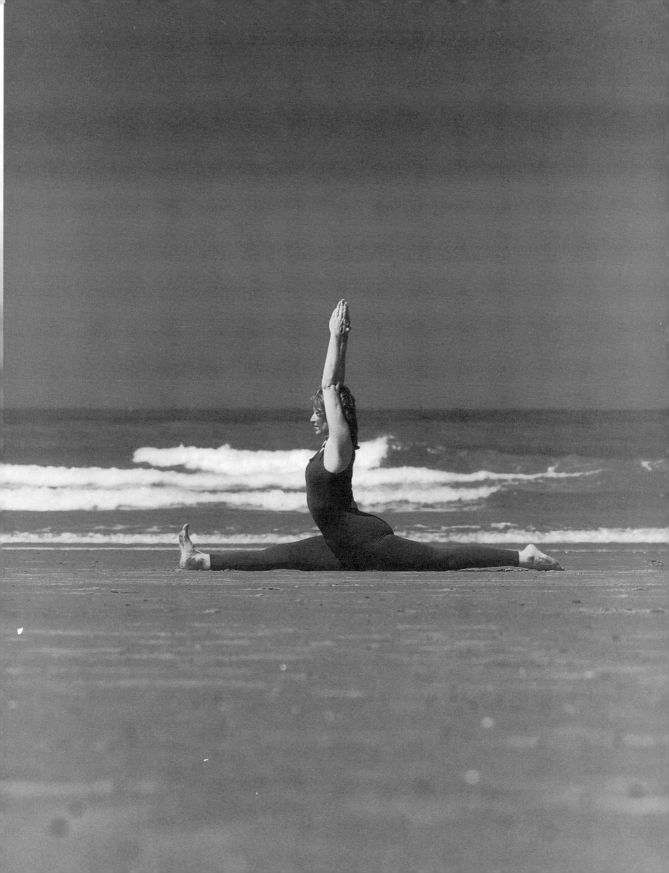

COOL

YOGA

TRICKS

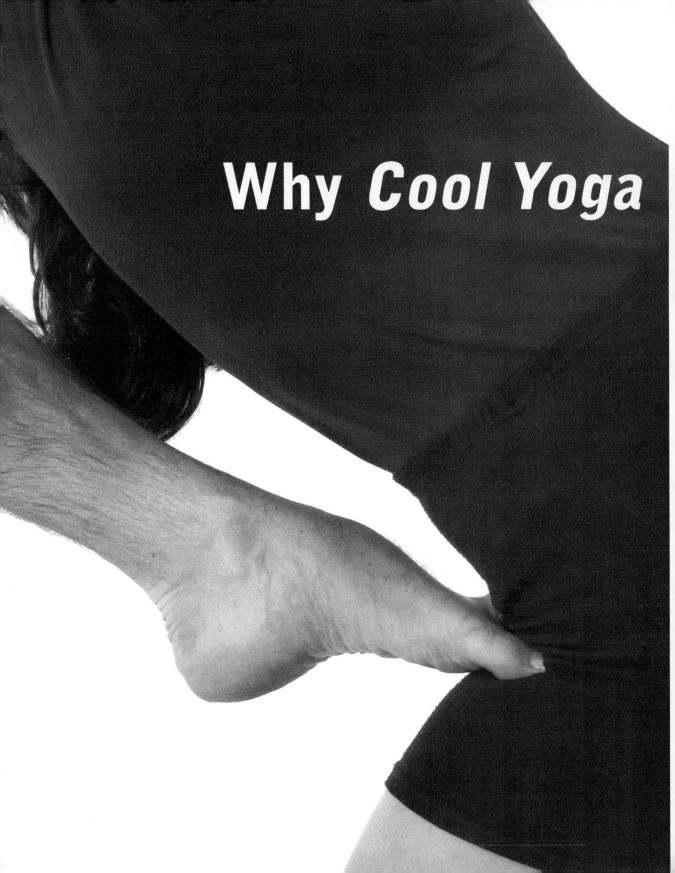

Why *Cool Yoga*

Tricks?

The reason millions of people are practicing yoga is that yoga gives us a sense of freedom and expansiveness in our bodies, minds, and spirits. This sense of freedom is different from the endorphin high that people experience in Western exercise. As various poses are mastered, the practitioner experiences enhanced self-esteem—a sense of mastery of his world. Strength-building poses give us a sense of both internal and external strength, and as we become more flexible in our bodies, we become more flexible in our attitudes. Inversions help us find our internal balance and poise when our lives are upside down. Back bends open our hearts with love and compassion for ourselves and for others.

Practicing yoga poses leads to a much quieter mind. Internal mind chatter is what causes stress, and as that diminishes we have many more internal resources to offer to ourselves and to others. Ultimately, yoga practice leads to a completely quiet mind, which all spiritual traditions claim is the experience of God and/or the experience of our own divine nature.

While millions are practicing yoga, most people are physically unable to perform the "classic" poses. It can take many years of practice to acquire the strength, flexibility, and body awareness to perform some of the most basic yoga postures correctly. Yet, the more closely we can duplicate the classic poses, the more freedom and expansiveness we feel. This is one reason people stay interested in yoga—there is always an opportunity to improve their postures. And accordingly, always the opportunity to feel more alive and more connected to themselves, to others, and to the cosmos.

In light of that, this book is geared to the "beyond beginner, but far from accomplished" student; to preintermediate and intermediate practitioners.

Cool Yoga Tricks contains more than 200 tricks that involve the use of props—yoga mats, straps, blocks, blankets, chairs, and walls—to enhance your yoga practice. By employing these tricks, you will be able to move more fully into postures and enhance your sense of physical and spiritual freedom. Through the tricks, you will experience that "*ah-ha*" feeling that comes from performing the postures in the manner that is most correct for your body.

While all of the techniques in *Cool Yoga Tricks* will improve your ability to perform yoga poses more easily and effortlessly, the tricks specifically assist in:

- bringing an enhanced feeling of freedom in your body and spirit

- increasing flexibility, strength, and endurance

- lengthening your spine and back muscles more completely

- strengthening back muscles, which can bring a permanent end to back problems

- opening your hips more fully, which also eases back pain

- releasing the neck and shoulder muscles, allowing healing of neck pain

- expanding awareness

- improving concentration

- allowing practice of certain postures if you are injured, ill, or overly tired

- healing injuries

- improving circulation

- enhancing relaxation at the end of your practice

- quieting your mind

As you read through this book and try the various postures, allow your body to guide you.

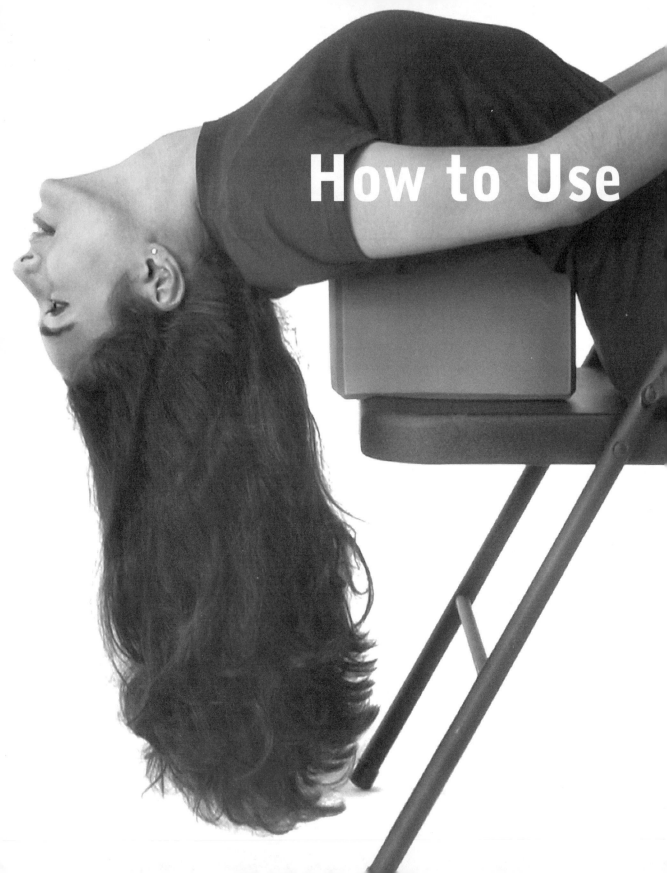

How to Use

the Tricks

At the beginning of each chapter is a brief discussion of the category of postures presented. Within the chapter, many classic or traditional yoga poses are depicted, with detailed instructions on how to enter the pose and suggested alignment adjustments to make while in the pose. The tricks that help you learn how to master these traditional postures follow. The book is organized this way because prior to practicing the suggested tricks, it is necessary to understand the most important components of each classic pose. Each trick helps you assimilate a certain aspect or aspects of the traditional posture.

You have learned the fundamentals of most of these poses in your yoga class or from a favorite book or tape. Perhaps what you have learned about some poses is different from what is presented here. That is because there are often many different ways to practice any given pose. There is no right or wrong way to do a pose. One variation may give one person more freedom in the pose, while another person may feel more constricted. That is largely due to our unique skeletal structure, musculature, and any injuries or illnesses we may be nursing.

Some of the suggested adjustments may surprise you. At first you may be doubtful of whether you can do them or skeptical as to whether they will make a difference. The best way to determine if a variation or alignment suggestion is right for you is to try it. Let your body be the judge. As you experiment with a particular aspect of the pose, be completely aware of your body. How do you feel while in a particular variation? Does the trick give you more freedom in your body or less? Do you feel more alertness in your body or your mind? Are you more relaxed in the pose even though you may be working harder than you normally do? Do you feel stronger and more flexible in the pose? And, consequently, do you find other poses easier?

It is important to let your body be your guide. Yoga awakens the body's intelligence and as you continue to practice, you become more and more discerning as to what is right and what is wrong for you and what meets your individual needs. Trust your body, trust your intuition, and trust yourself.

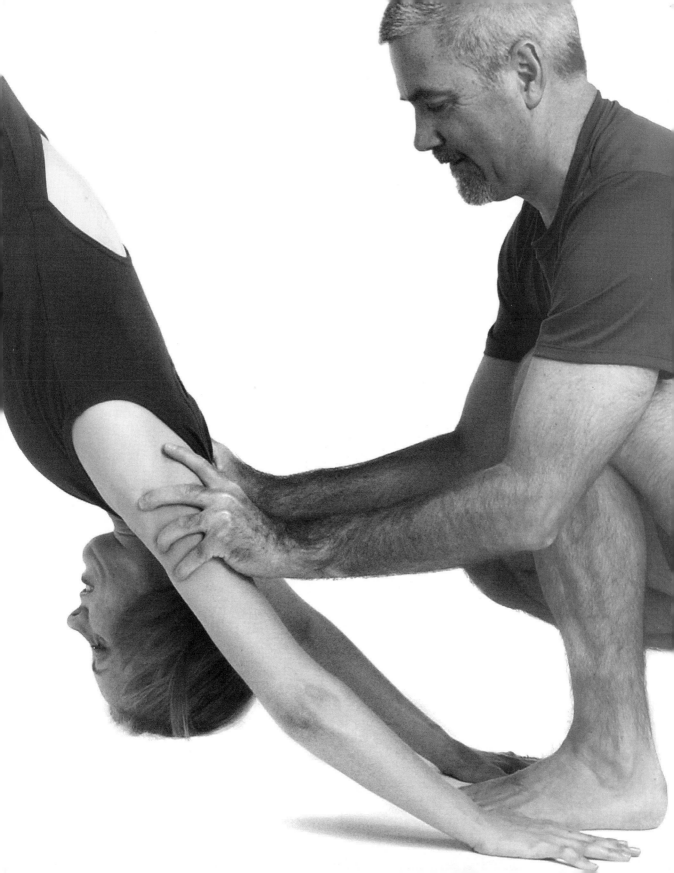

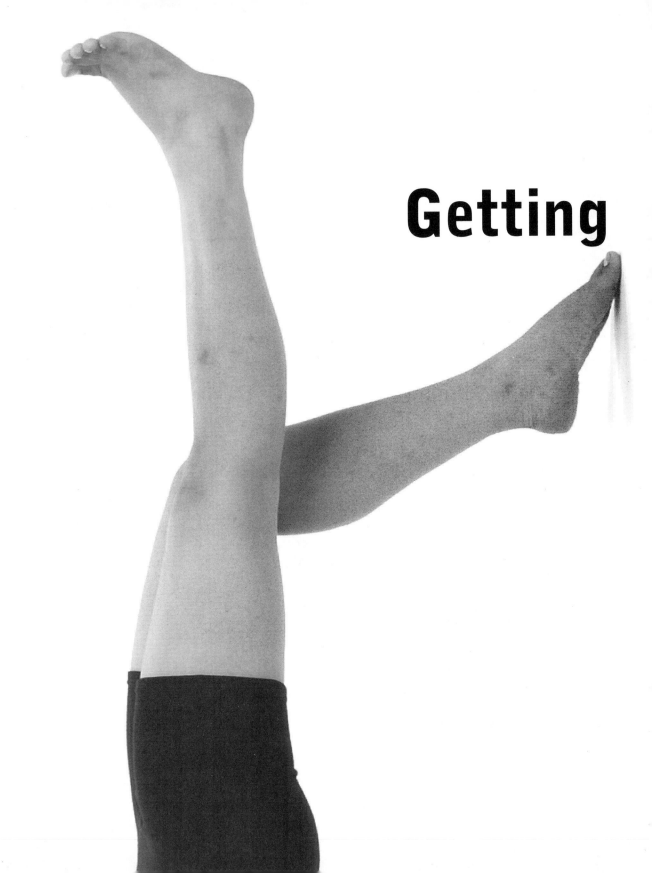

Getting

Started

This book is designed for beginner, beyond-beginner, preintermediate, and intermediate yoga students. As a reader, then, you are familiar with most of the postures that are presented here. You have probably performed many of these postures in your yoga classes or at home, using a video or book. What may be new to you are the alignment instructions and the use of props to assist your alignment. This section will help you get acquainted with the props and some of the primary alignment instructions.

STANDARD TRICKS

As you read through this book and practice the tricks, you will notice that there is continuity to the alignment directions. Alignment instructions are repeated in the various poses and in the various categories of poses. Some of the alignment cues given for standing poses, for example, are duplicated for forward bends, back bends, and inversions. Perfecting the alignment techniques in the simpler poses makes performing the more difficult postures easier.

This chapter includes some of the primary tricks to help you learn the most common alignment techniques. The alignment instructions for each posture will come later, sometimes with reference to the tricks in this chapter and at other times presented in new ways that are most appropriate for a particular posture. My advice is to practice some of these movements prior to performing them in postures. That way, you will gain a deeper understanding, which will make them easier to execute in the poses.

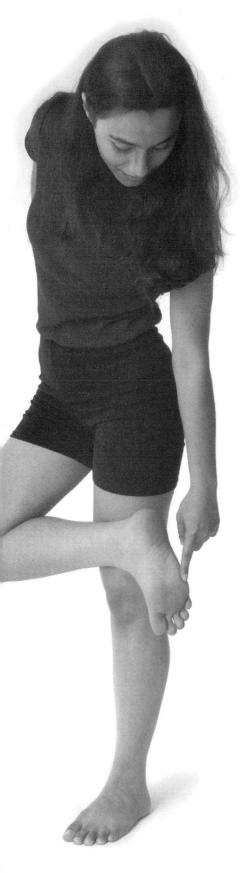

Primary Tricks

The Four Corners of the Feet—a Note About the Importance of Feet

The feet are the foundation of our bodies. How we position our feet affects our whole body, and particularly our legs, hips, and lower back. As such, activating our feet properly is of utmost importance in any yoga posture.

In standing poses, we stand on our feet. In back bends we firmly position our feet so we don't falter while in a vulnerable position. In inversions, we stretch our feet toward the ceiling, helping to stabilize the legs and the lower back.

Standing with proper foot placement, with equal weight on both feet, and with a heightened awareness of our feet is a good place to start. The first yogic standing pose is Samasthithi, or "Equal Standing" in English. (It is also known as Tadasana, or Mountain Pose.) To stand equally, think about each foot having four corners. Two of the corners are located at the top of the heel, on the inside and outside edges. The other two corners are found at the bottom of the ball of the foot, again at the inside and outside edges.

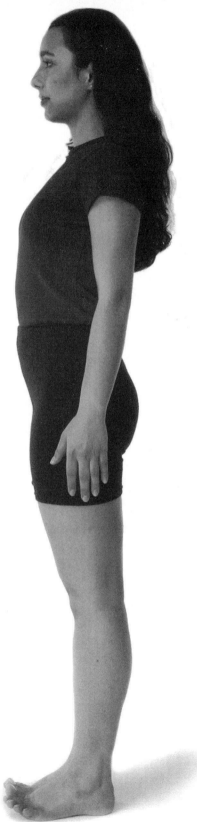

To activate your awareness of these corners, place your finger on each corner. Then, to understand how to stand on these corners, stand in Samasthithi. Lift the ball of your right foot and slowly place the inside edge of the ball of the foot on the floor. Then, with equal awareness, place the outside edge of the ball of your foot on the floor. Repeat this process with the left foot.

Then, lift your right heel. Slowly and consciously, place the inside and then the outside edge of your heel on the floor. Repeat with your left heel. With full awareness, feel the four corners pressing into the floor.

If you can't quite feel them, lift your toes, which will allow you to feel them more fully. Make sure that you are distributing your weight equally, that you are not placing more of your weight on one foot or on your heels or the balls of your feet.

Bring this increased awareness of the placement of your feet to all of your standing poses. Deliberately press the four corners of your feet into the floor. Do the same in your back-bend practice. In forward bends, stretch the four corners of the feet away from you, and in inversions, press the four corners of the feet toward the ceiling. In your daily life, even when wearing shoes, practice pressing the four corners of your feet into the ground. Do so when you are walking or standing still. This increased awareness will benefit your yoga practice and the way you feel in general, making you feel more balanced and grounded.

Lifting and Rolling the Thighs

"Lift the thighs" is an alignment instruction that you will find in many categories of poses—standing postures, forward bends, and inversions. In other words, lift your quadriceps, the muscles on the front of the thighs, toward your hips.

Other terminology that I use to help get this point across includes:

- engage the thighs or engage the quadriceps

- contract the thighs or contract the quadriceps

This direction can be confusing and elusive for many students. Even for me. In fact, after the first class in which I finally got it, I was so proud of myself that I went home and spent the next several hours lifting my thighs.

Another alignment direction that is often combined with the instruction of "lift your thighs" is "roll your thighs inward" or "roll your thighs outward." Here are some tricks that will help you learn to lift, engage, or contract your thighs and roll them inward or outward. In forward bends and inversions, we are normally taught to roll the thighs inward. In some standing poses, the thighs roll outward; in others, the thighs roll inward. And, as one would expect in yoga, in other standing poses the instruction is to roll one thigh outward and the other thigh inward.

Rolling in specific directions or in opposite directions seems crazy—even impossible—to those who are new to yoga. Yet there is a reason for this seeming madness, which becomes overwhelmingly apparent once we can actualize the movements. When our thighs are rolled appropriately, our spines align and we feel an exciting new sense of freedom in our bodies.

LIFTING AND ROLLING THE THIGHS INWARD

- Place a yoga block between your thighs, as high as possible, and bring your feet as close together as you can.

- Adjust yourself in Samasthithi. Feel the four corners of each foot.

- The block naturally lifts/contracts/engages your quadriceps, which is the next alignment instruction given for Samasthithi.

- Lift your lower back and abdomen, which is made easier with the block.

- Lift your sternum. Soften the tops of your shoulders, neck, throat, and face.

- In Samasthithi, the alignment instruction is to roll your thighs inward. Gently push the block behind you. This "overdoes" the action but it gives your body the memory of how to roll your thighs inward when you are not using the block.

- Notice that when your quads are lifted and rolling inward, your lower back and lower abdomen lift effortlessly. This also allows your entire spine to straighten more easily.

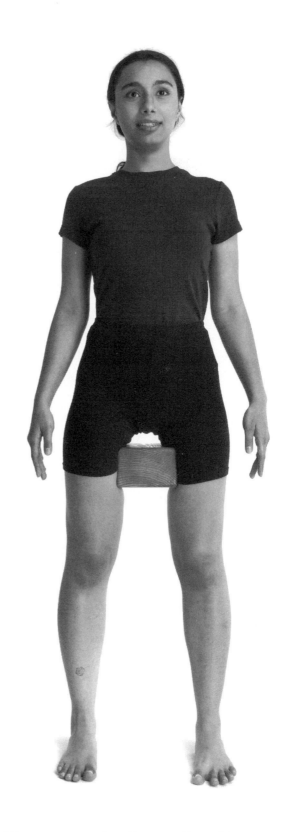

LIFTING AND ROLLING THE THIGHS OUTWARD

- Stand in the prepose position for Triangle or Warrior II—feet separated by about four feet, with the right foot turned out ninety degrees, and the left foot turned slightly in toward the right foot.

- Bend your forward knee slightly.

- As you straighten it, engage your quads and roll your thigh outward.

- Then slightly bend the knee of your back leg, and as you straighten it, lift your quads and roll the thigh outward.

- Concentrate on maintaining the lift and outward rotation throughout the pose. It is easy to release them if you are not mindful.

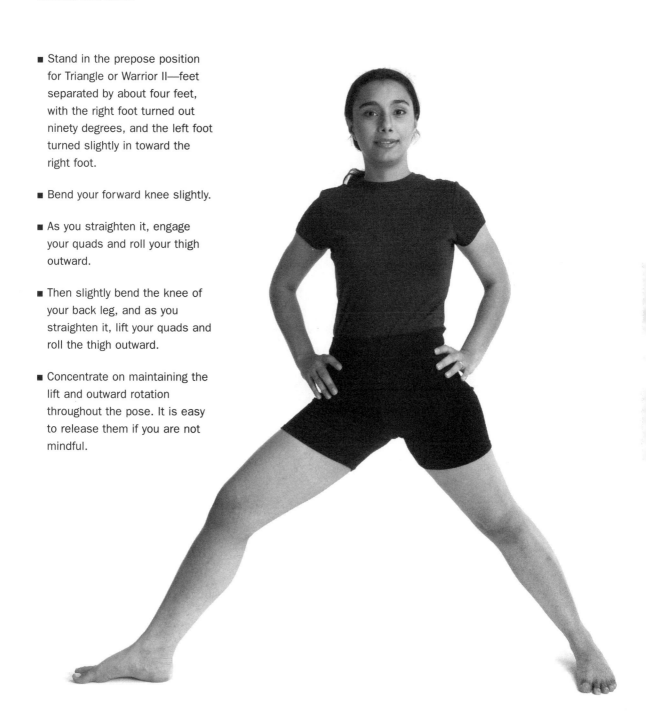

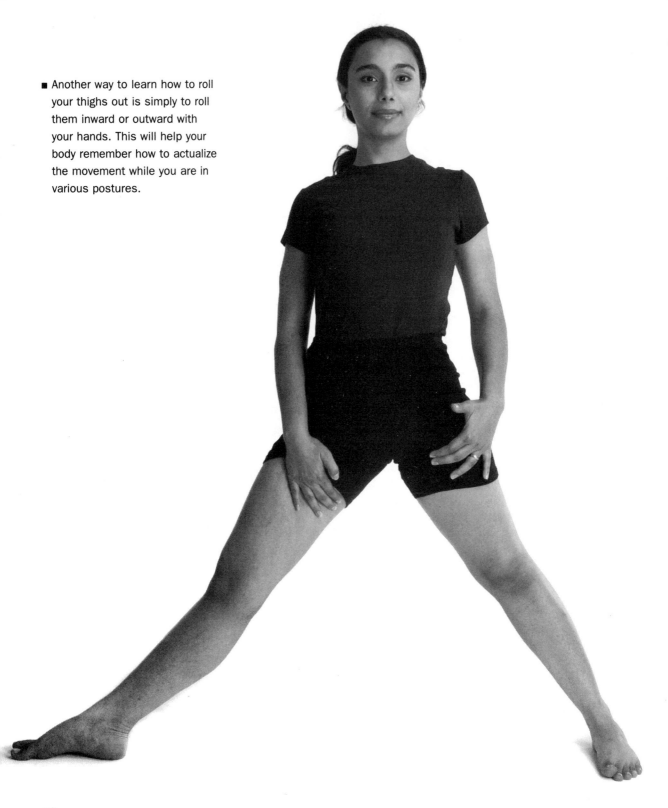

■ Another way to learn how to roll your thighs out is simply to roll them inward or outward with your hands. This will help your body remember how to actualize the movement while you are in various postures.

Ground the Femur Bones, or Press the Fronts of the Thighs Toward the Backs of the Thighs

"Ground the femur bones" (thighbones) is another alignment instruction that is consistent in standing poses, forward bends, and inversions. To clarify that instruction, I often say, "Press the fronts of your thighs toward the backs of your thighs." I particularly use that phrase in Downward-Facing Dog. No matter how it is articulated, the following trick can help you master the action.

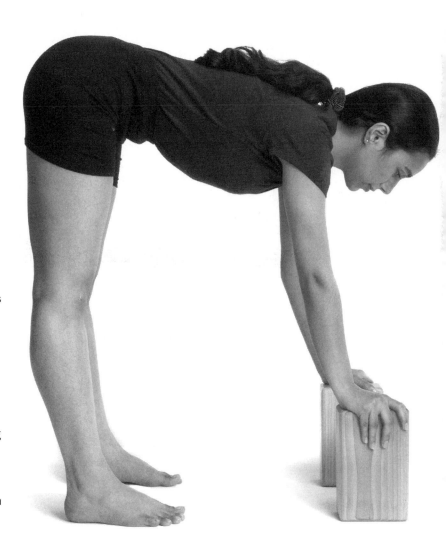

- Stand two blocks at their highest height about twelve inches in front of you. Your feet and legs should be hip-distance apart.

- From the hip crease, lean forward and place your hands on the blocks.

- In this posture, press the fronts of your thighs toward the backs of your thighs. Notice how much easier the action is in this posture than when you try it while standing upright.

- Allow your body's intelligence to remember this action when you try it in other poses.

Shoulder-Alignment Cues

In working the arms and shoulders in many postures—
Downward Dog, back bends, and inversions—a common alignment instruction is "Roll the outside edge of your armpits and
deltoid muscles

■ forward,

■ outward, or

■ toward the floor."

The action is the same, but the instruction varies depending on
what position your are in. The idea is to roll the outside edges of
your armpits and deltoid muscles away from your body. An easy
way to learn how to manipulate your armpits enough to roll
them is to practice the following instructions by yourself or get a
friend to help you.

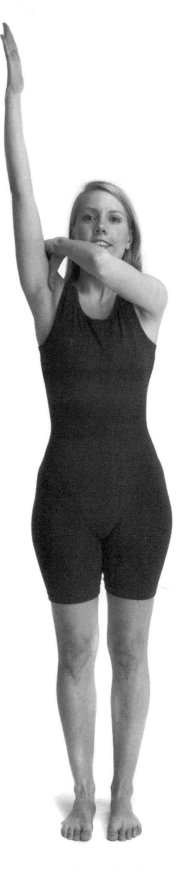

■ If you are doing this yourself,
raise one arm overhead with
your palm facing inward.

■ With the opposite hand, grab
the deltoid muscle and roll it in
the direction away from your
body.

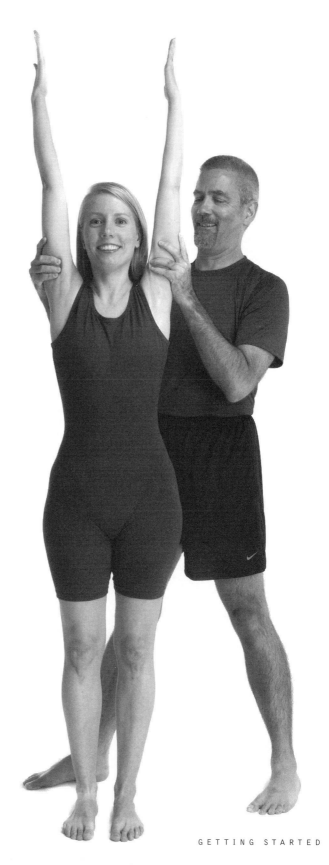

■ Alternatively, raise both arms with your palms facing each other. Have a friend stand behind you and roll your deltoid muscles away from your body.

■ Feel the sensation and try to duplicate it in the postures in which you see the instruction.

TAPE METHOD OF ARM ROLLING

Okay, it is easy enough to roll your armpits and deltoids when somebody does it for you. "But how do I do that on my own?" you ask. Here's the answer: use athletic tape to roll your deltoids away from your body prior to a session in which you will be practicing many postures that require this action.

Use athletic tape that is three inches wide. I particularly like Elastikon tape, which is made by Johnson & Johnson. (Yes, this is a plug.) I have tried many brands and this is my favorite. It is flexible enough to allow movement and firm enough to keep your deltoids where you want them. So get your tape and a pair of scissors and start rolling.

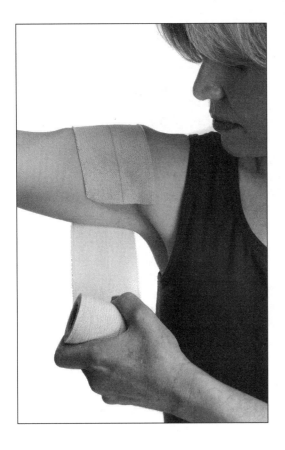

If possible, have a friend roll your upper arm outward—away from your body. If there is no friend to help you, when you secure the first part of the tape around your arm, firmly pull the tape outward, again away from your body.

Place the end of the tape at the very top of your arm near the shoulder joint and on the inside edge of your armpit. Cover the top of your arm and pull firmly, so your muscles are turning outward (away from your body). Continue this procedure, particularly the part where you pull the muscles outward. Tape until you have covered the upper arm about two inches above your elbow.

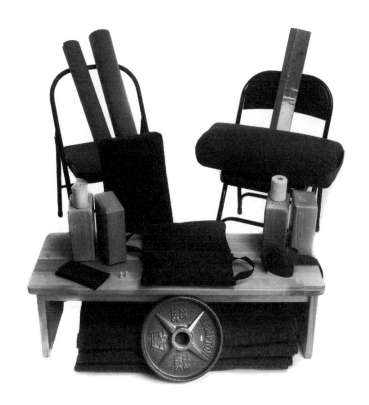

THE USE OF PROPS

Yogacharya B.K.S. Iyengar introduced the use of props to help people who otherwise could not perform a particular pose assume the posture—and more important, assume the posture in a way that is most beneficial for their specific needs. For many years Iyengar was chided as the "furniture yogi." As yoga has become more popular, the use of props has become widespread. When I started practicing yoga in the mid-1980s, the production and sale of yoga props was basically a small, home-based business: one guy in the class would make some blocks and benches and sell them to other students. Occasionally there was a woman who made eye bags and sandbags. Straps had to be imported from India. Good yoga mats were difficult to obtain. Now, yoga-prop mail-order catalogs are a thriving business, and many national retail chains sell packages of yoga props. How times change!

Props allow people to assume postures that are right for their bodies. In some cases, the props make the pose more difficult because you are doing the posture correctly. Though you may be working harder with the prop, you will notice an increased sense of openness, freedom, and/or relaxation in your body.

Necessary Props

As you know, your yoga mat is basic to your practice. Although I prefer to do most of my postures on a hardwood floor, a yoga mat is necessary for carpeted areas and for many specific poses. *Note: All yoga mats are not created equal.* Some of the packages of props that are sold by retail chains include mats that are shorter and narrower than the standard mat. More important, many mats do not adhere to carpeted surfaces and can slip, possibly causing a fall and an injury. (Unfortunately, I'm all too familiar with this problem.) So make sure you really do have a nonslip or "sticky" mat. In fact, I recommend having at least two of them.

Yoga straps are fairly standard. I personally prefer the metal fasteners to the plastic ones.

Wooden blocks work for all poses, and I prefer them. Yet when I teach at studios other than my own, I am amazed that foam blocks actually work just fine for most poses. Foam blocks can get a little squishy in some poses. Yet for other postures they are better than wooden blocks. Choose the type of block you prefer, and if possible, have two of each.

Sturdy blankets are most appropriate for yoga practice. Department-store blankets are fine for sitting on in forward bends or for restorative back bends, but they are not firm enough for inversions. So when you are ready for headstands and shoulder stands, get some sturdy blankets. Wool or cotton is best.

Metal folding chairs are good for many postures. Be sure to get one that is sturdy. Shop around a little bit; some national chains carry lightweight chairs that can tip over when your weight is unevenly distributed on them, as it often is in yoga. The heavier ones are more reliable. Some people like the backless chairs, which can usually be found only in yoga supply catalogs.

Hand towels or face cloths can be useful for some poses. Have a couple in your yoga kit.

Perhaps the most important prop is one that is not sold in yoga supply catalogs, but I am sure you have one at home. It is a wall. Make sure you have one bare wall in the room where you practice your poses. Caution: your wall is likely to get footprints and handprints on it over time—a visible tribute to your hard work!

Optional Props

There are many optional props that can make your yoga practice a delight. For example, I particularly favor using a Setu Bandha bench for supported Setu Bandha, but you will see that there are many other ways to practice the pose with other props that you probably already have on hand. These benches can also be used for other postures, but again, other props can be substituted.

Halasana benches are terrific, but they have only one purpose. Because a chair can be substituted for them in that one pose, Supported Halasana (Plow Pose), we demonstrate the pose that way.

Bolsters are normally used for restorative postures. However, in most cases, blankets can be rolled and used in place of bolsters. But bolsters are so convenient to grab and lie over quickly at the end of a stressful day.

Slant boards are great for grounding your back heel in some standing poses, and lifting your wrist in Downward Dog and in some inversions and back bends. But folded yoga mats usually work just as well. There is one truly awesome trick in which a slant board is used in Revolved Triangle. I have not tried a smooth two-by-four but my bet is that it works just as well.

Eye covers and earplugs are great for restorative postures and final relaxation. I personally don't think I could live without them.

As stated earlier, I use athletic tape to help my deltoids roll outward. I also use it sometimes (more in my earlier days of yoga practice than now) to tape my wrists to give me more support for back bends, handstands, Downward Dog, Plank Pose, and Sun Salutations.

A FEW WORDS OF CAUTION

■ Move into the poses slowly, deliberately, and with full awareness of your movements. Do not be in a hurry to get into or out
of the poses.

■ Remember to breathe continuously, smoothly, and evenly. It is
easy to stop breathing when we are challenged. In some poses,
breathing naturally becomes difficult. This is why it is important to remind ourselves to breathe smoothly and evenly.

■ Detailed alignment instructions for individual poses are given
next to each classic or traditional posture. The classic postures
are the ones photographed outside. The tricks for each posture
follow. With many of the tricks, I do not repeat all of the alignment cues, but you should refer back to them as needed. In
addition to some of the standard tricks given on the previous
few pages, I want to remind you of some basics.

1. In many postures it is important to lengthen your spine as
   much as you can. This creates more space and freedom in the
   body and nourishes the spinal system through improved circulation. Lengthening the spine can normally be accomplished by lifting the lower back and lower abdomen, and
   your sternum. If you round your back, except where explic-
   itly directed, you will train your spine to curve.

2. Lengthening the spine does not mean lifting your shoulders
   toward your ears, which must be a natural physiological
   response because so many of us do that as beginners.
   Consciously soften the tops of your shoulders when you lift
   your sternum or your spine.

3. Keep your throat, neck, jaw, and face relaxed.

4. In many forward bends and standing postures, keep your

head aligned with your spine. In other words, do not tilt your head forward or backward (the most common error) or to one side or the other. If you do, you will simply get a neck ache and blame yoga.

5. I recommend moving from the "hip crease" in most of the forward bends and in some standing postures. The hip crease is the hip joint, the place where the top of the thigh and the pelvis meet.

6. Inversions should not be practiced during menses.

7. If you have an injury or illness, discuss the problem and your yoga practice with your doctor. Modify your poses according to his or her recommendations. Refer to page 28 about yoga injuries.

OTHER THINGS TO REMEMBER

Many beginning students have a love-hate relationship with yoga. At times, practicing yoga can be difficult. At other times, it exhilarates us. If you are not in the mood to practice yoga, try a few poses anyway. Sometimes if you do, you will then feel like doing more. If after a few poses you still don't want to practice, quit and try again another day.

If you want to practice but don't have the time, practice for five minutes. Everybody has five extra minutes. Ten minutes, maybe not, but everybody has five minutes to spare. A little yoga is better than no yoga.

The most important part of a yoga practice is to enjoy it. If you are not having fun, not feeling better as a result of doing yoga, or you are generally miserable—choose a different discipline.

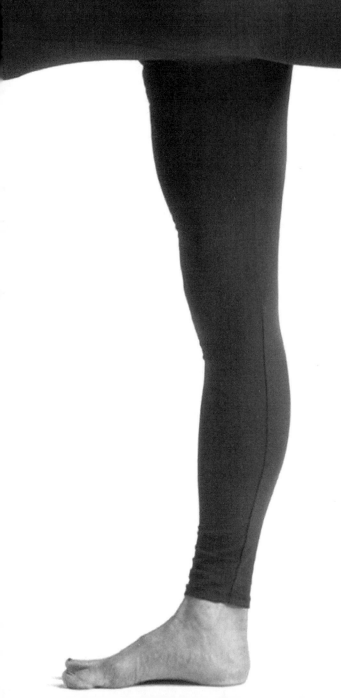

A Word About

Injuries

Doing yoga on a regular basis is known as yoga practice. And because it is a practice, you don't have to be perfect. Yoga is about working with your own body at your own level. Be gentle and compassionate with yourself, and with your body. Do not force your body into a pose for which it is not ready. Doing so leads to misalignment and possibly to injury.

This is why there are many options for each pose. Choose the variation that works for you *now*. Over time you can graduate to an alternative pose. But remember that just because one alternative looks more demanding or interesting, if you are performing that variation incorrectly it will not give you the results you are seeking.

I tend to be very cautious with my students, maybe overly cautious. Indeed, we teach what we need to learn. I have had many injuries from yoga—both by pushing myself too hard and by teachers pushing me too hard. My bet is that there are many other yoga students like me. I have made all of the mistakes and am now advising others against making them.

My sense of competitiveness may be too finely honed. I have often tried poses I was not ready for because other people in the class were doing them. Sometimes performing the poses brought new awareness; other times I hurt myself. When I have had injuries, I have often thought, Oh, if I practice that pose, I will build strength in that area. Wrong! On one occasion, when I thought an injury had healed, I failed to tell a workshop teacher about it. Invariably, the teacher adjusted one of my poses in a way that reinjured me. That reinjury took several years to fully heal. Another time, I took the advice of a teacher who told me that if I worked through my shoulder pain, it would go away. The pain got worse. I then went to another teacher who told me the same thing. I continued the practice. Finally, my shoulder hurt so badly that I had to stop. Soon thereafter my shoulder completely froze and I was unable to practice any yoga at all for many months.

Injuries are not fun. It took many years, but I have finally learned to protect myself. I listen to my body's wisdom instead of my ego. I consider the teacher's advice, but also rational alternatives. It is not worth risking our health to do something that looks cool. It is important to resist our natural sense of competitiveness, which might drive us to do something that may hurt us. It is important to remember that underneath our skin is a complex system of muscles, ligaments, tendons, bones, organs, glands, arteries, veins, and nerves. We don't want to abuse these delicate systems on a whim. Please consider my advice: It is better to err on the side of caution than to go into a pose, or further into a pose, than you should.

Yoga can be a tricky balance. We are encouraged by teachers—and we ourselves want—to go beyond our limitations. Yet we also want to make realistic choices. Yoga is meant to bring us into the present moment. If we are truly present and attentive in the moment, we can make clear decisions about what pose is right for our body at this point in our practice. Maybe the thing we most need from yoga practice *in this moment* is the easier option. We can think of yoga as an exploration of our abilities and limitations. Understanding limitations, without going beyond them, is a worthy consideration.

With all of that said, I should also say that I do not regret my injuries. In fact, I have learned much more about the deeper aspects of yoga when I have been injured. One of the primary goals of yoga is to use the postures to quiet the mind, which leads to meditation. Yoga and meditation lead to the development of an inner peace that includes a deeper understanding of oneself and others. This inner peace can bring insights into the mystery of life, experiences of God. This inner peace is genuine happiness. As we experience it, we become more sensitive to others and are truly able to have more love and compassion for our fellow man.

When I have had injuries, I have learned to be more present in my poses, and my practice of postures has become more meditative. Consequently, my mind has become quieter. During these phases, I have learned how to work with students who have similar injuries and have become a better teacher by understanding their pain, frustration, and limitations.

Admittedly, during recuperation times, I have whined and felt sorry for myself. When that phase has passed, I have turned my attention to people who have had injuries (not self-induced) more serious than mine. When injured, I have meditated more and practiced meditations specifically designed to develop compassion. By concentrating on the pain of others—the pain of people who are hungry, homeless, truly sick, or injured—I have been able to get out of my egocentric self just a little bit more.

Yoga is ultimately not about wrapping our legs around our necks or arching back into beautiful back bends. It is about using the body as an instrument to fully realize and stay connected to our own inner joy, love, and compassion. Yoga is about opening our hearts with love and compassion to others who suffer in innumerable ways. Yoga is not about touching our toes. It is about tenderly touching the hearts of the people around us.

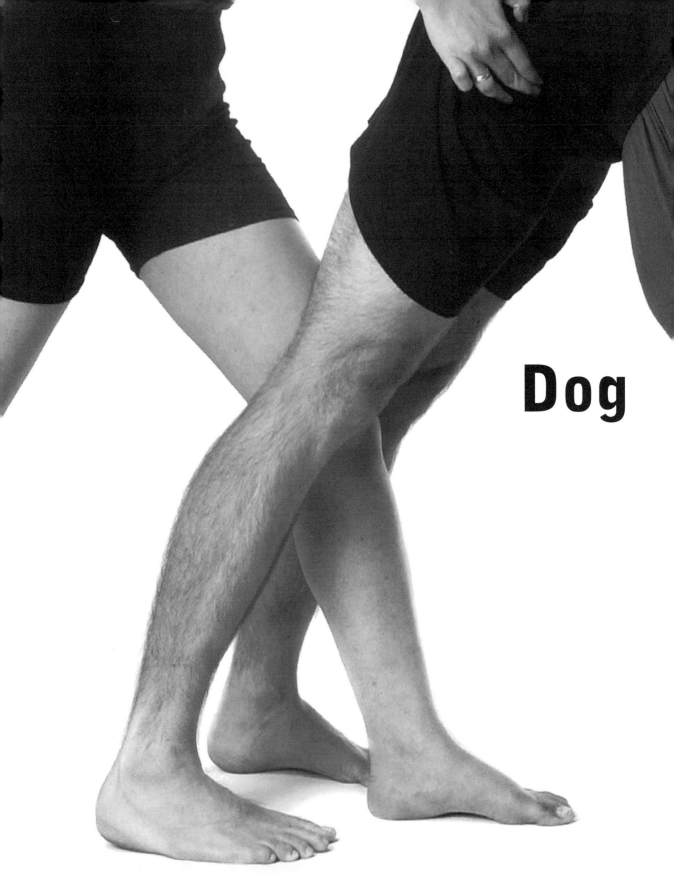

Dog

Tricks

Perhaps you've seen the T-shirts—*Another Day, Another Dog Pose*—expressing the drudgery we all sometimes feel about Downward Dog. There can be no doubt, Downward-Facing Dog can be difficult and tiring, especially for beginning yoga students. Yet, for many of us, beginners as well as advanced students, it is our first pose of the day. And it is usually our most-often-practiced pose. Why? It's the all-purpose pose. It builds strength and flexibility in the arms, shoulders, back, and legs. The tension in our backs and our necks melts away. It makes us feel alive, alert, strong, and centered. From Dog, other poses flow easily.

When practicing Dog, we experience the most lightness when our form is precise—or most attuned to our own individual needs and abilities. This chapter is dedicated to getting the most out of your Dog. It gives a variety of techniques to help you extend your spine, relax your neck, strengthen your body, and increase your flexibility. When practicing the tricks presented in this chapter, your love for your Dog will magnify. With these tricks, Downward-Facing Dog will indeed become an "effortless effort." You will feel more alive, more stretched out, and more powerful in the pose—and you will look forward to *Another Day, Another Dog Pose.*

ADHO MUKHA SVANASANA
Downward-Facing Dog

There are a couple of standard ways to get into Dog Pose. The pose is often assumed by kneeling on all fours, with your hands shoulder-distance apart and your feet hip-distance apart. Concave your lower back, straighten your knees—leading with your sit bones. Another common way to get into the pose is from Uttanasana, Standing Forward Bend, in which you walk your hands and feet away from each other. Come into the pose in your favorite manner and then make the following adjustments.

- Your feet should be about four feet from your hands.

- Make sure your fingers are spread wide and that your palms are firmly pressing down into the floor.

- Your hands should be shoulder-distance apart and your feet should be hip-distance apart.

- Fully extend your arms and torso.

- Roll the outside edges of your armpits and your deltoid muscles toward the floor. This makes more space in the upper back and allows your neck to hang more freely, which releases the tension in your neck.

- Lift your quadriceps and roll them inward. Press the fronts of your thighs toward the backs of your thighs.

- Stretch the backs of your thighs toward your heels and work on pressing your heels into the floor.

- Press your forearms away from you and the insides of your elbows toward each other.

- Allow your head to hang toward the floor, with your neck muscles completely relaxed. If possible, allow the crown of your head to touch the floor.

- Practice in this way:

  - On your inhalation, extend your arms and your torso toward your hips. Roll your deltoids toward the floor and drop your head.

  - On your exhalation, press the fronts of your thighs toward the backs of your thighs, roll your thighs inward, and extend the backs of your thighs toward your heels and your heels toward the floor.

  - Continue in this manner until your movements become extremely subtle.

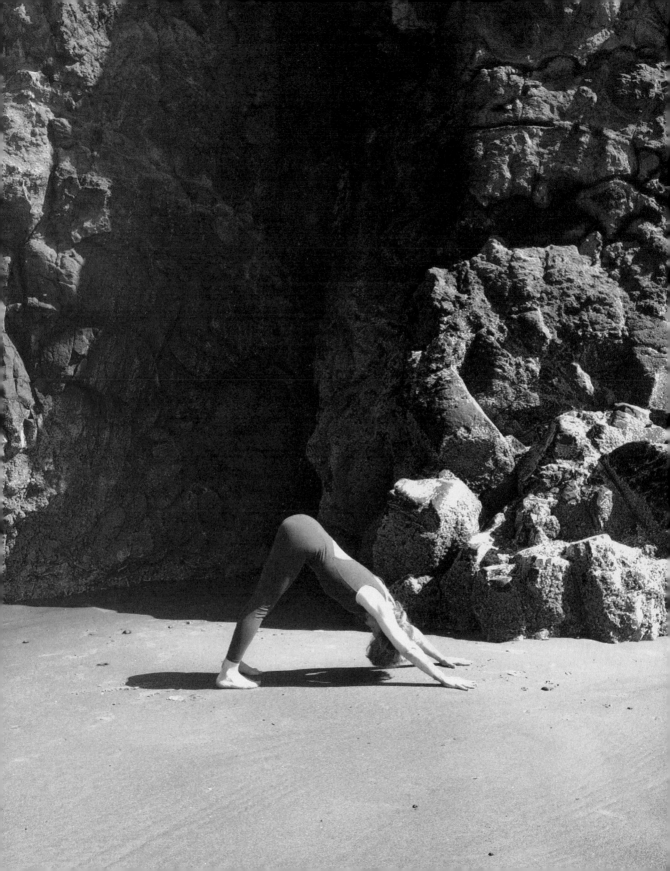

If you are tiring quickly in Downward-Facing Dog, it is probably because there is too much pressure on your arms and shoulders. The weight of the pose should rest in your legs and hips, which are stronger and less vulnerable to fatigue than your arms and shoulders. The key to bringing your weight back is fourfold:

- lifting your quadriceps muscles

- rolling your thighs inward

- pressing the fronts of your thighs toward the backs of your thighs

- lengthening your spine

You will find that the first three actions also lengthen your spine, giving you more overall extension in the pose. With the pressure off your arms and shoulders, you can work on the arm and shoulder movements:

- roll the outside edges of your armpits and deltoid muscles toward the floor

- press your elbows toward each other

- lift your wrist muscles toward your elbows

- press your forearms slightly forward

As you master these movements with the tricks in this chapter, you will find more lightness in your Dog Pose and more lightness in your spirit. Many of these tricks are self-explanatory. But be sure to use the alignment techniques given on page 34.

Assume the pose and have a friend pull the top of your thighs toward her.

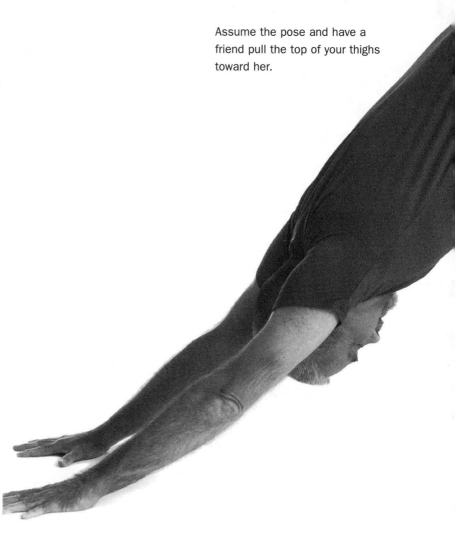

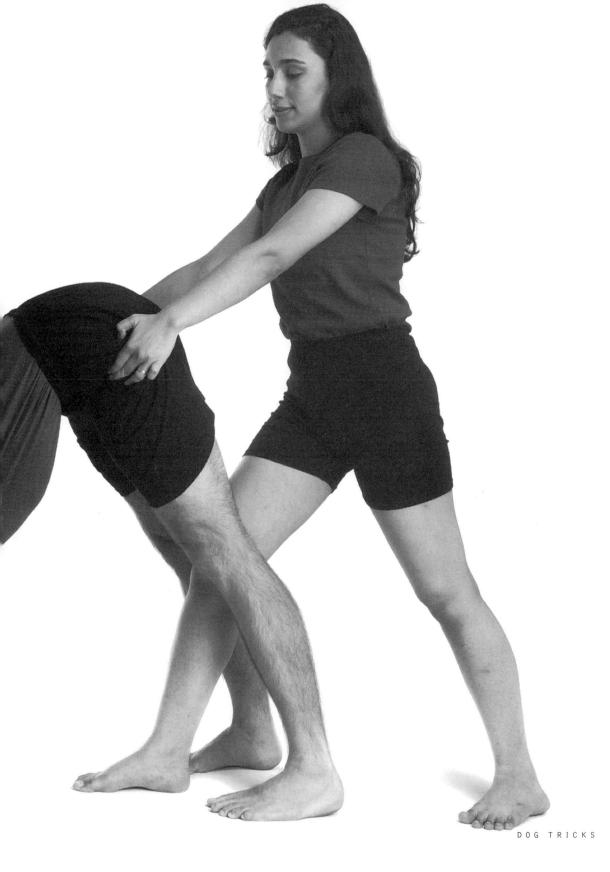

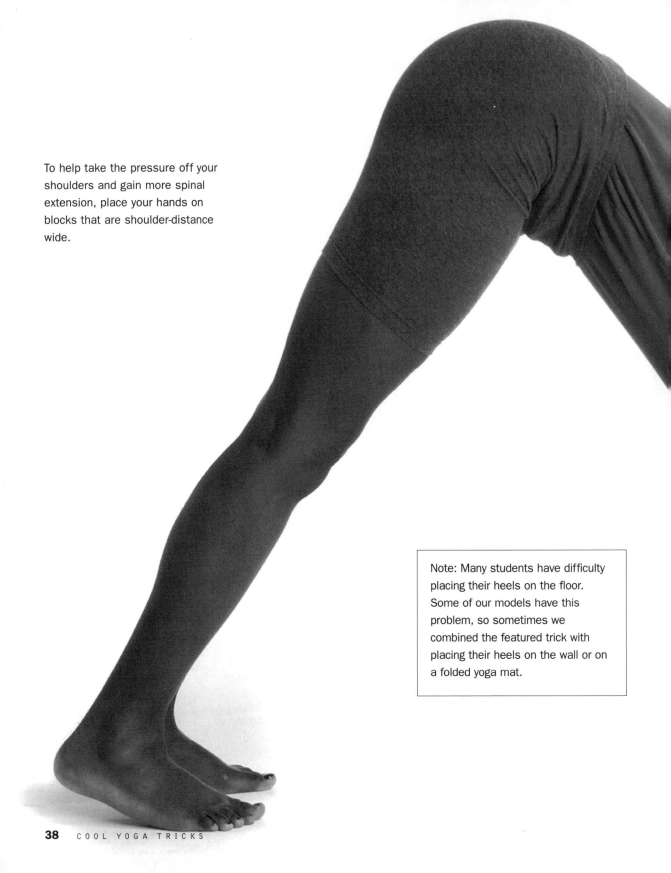

To help take the pressure off your shoulders and gain more spinal extension, place your hands on blocks that are shoulder-distance wide.

Note: Many students have difficulty placing their heels on the floor. Some of our models have this problem, so sometimes we combined the featured trick with placing their heels on the wall or on a folded yoga mat.

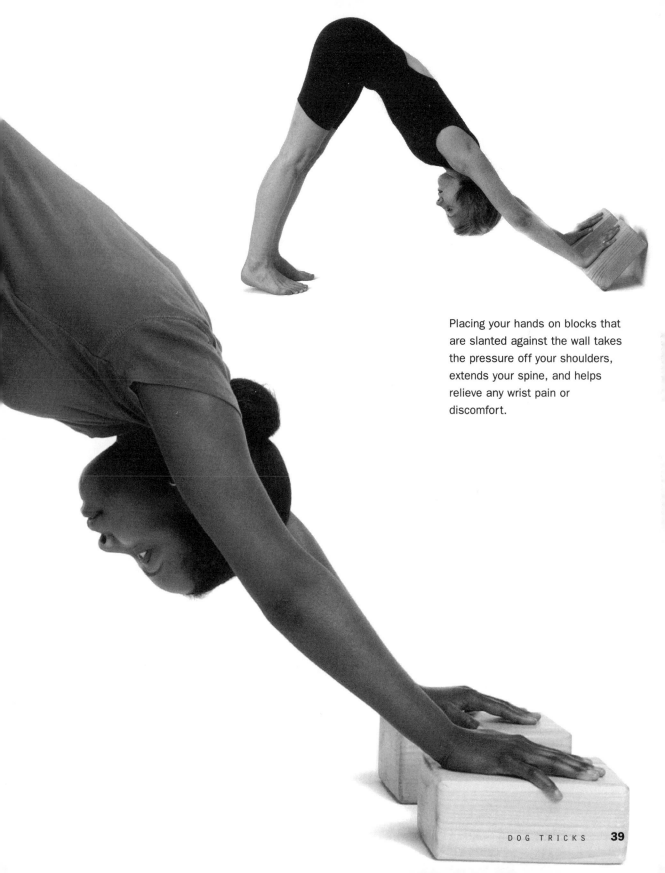

Placing your hands on blocks that are slanted against the wall takes the pressure off your shoulders, extends your spine, and helps relieve any wrist pain or discomfort.

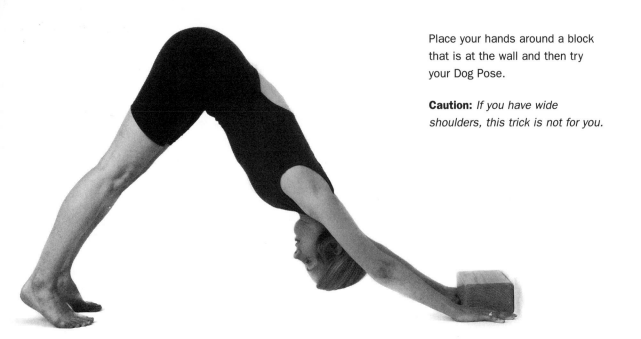

Place your hands around a block that is at the wall and then try your Dog Pose.

Caution: *If you have wide shoulders, this trick is not for you.*

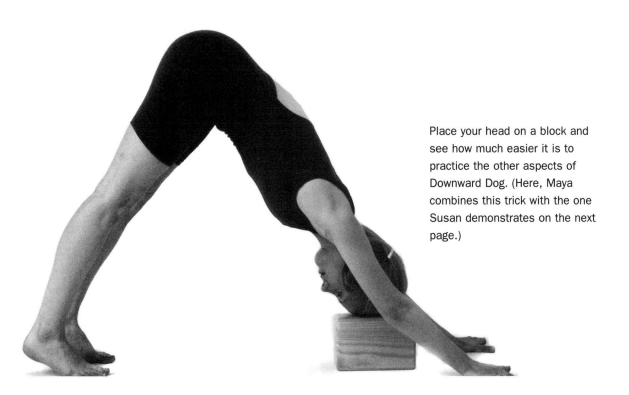

Place your head on a block and see how much easier it is to practice the other aspects of Downward Dog. (Here, Maya combines this trick with the one Susan demonstrates on the next page.)

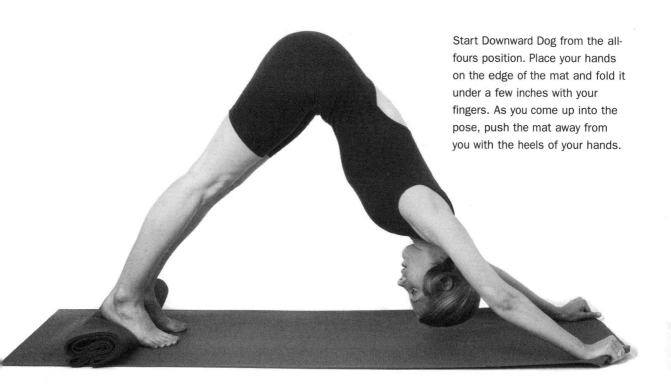

Start Downward Dog from the all-fours position. Place your hands on the edge of the mat and fold it under a few inches with your fingers. As you come up into the pose, push the mat away from you with the heels of your hands.

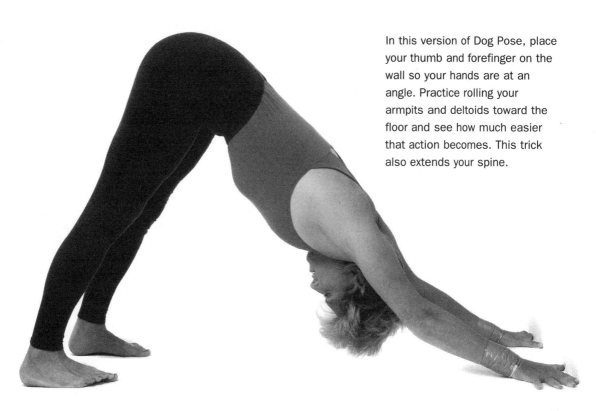

In this version of Dog Pose, place your thumb and forefinger on the wall so your hands are at an angle. Practice rolling your armpits and deltoids toward the floor and see how much easier that action becomes. This trick also extends your spine.

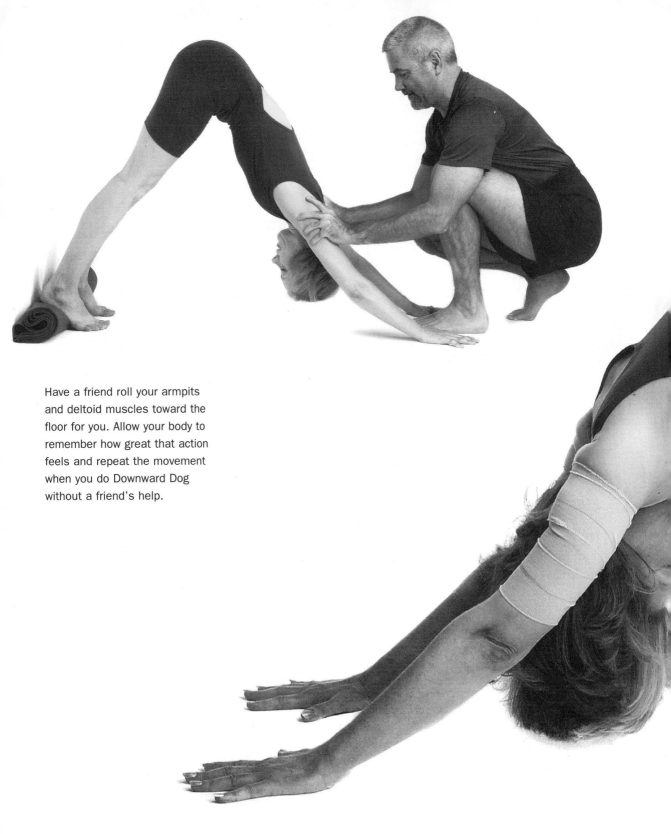

Have a friend roll your armpits and deltoid muscles toward the floor for you. Allow your body to remember how great that action feels and repeat the movement when you do Downward Dog without a friend's help.

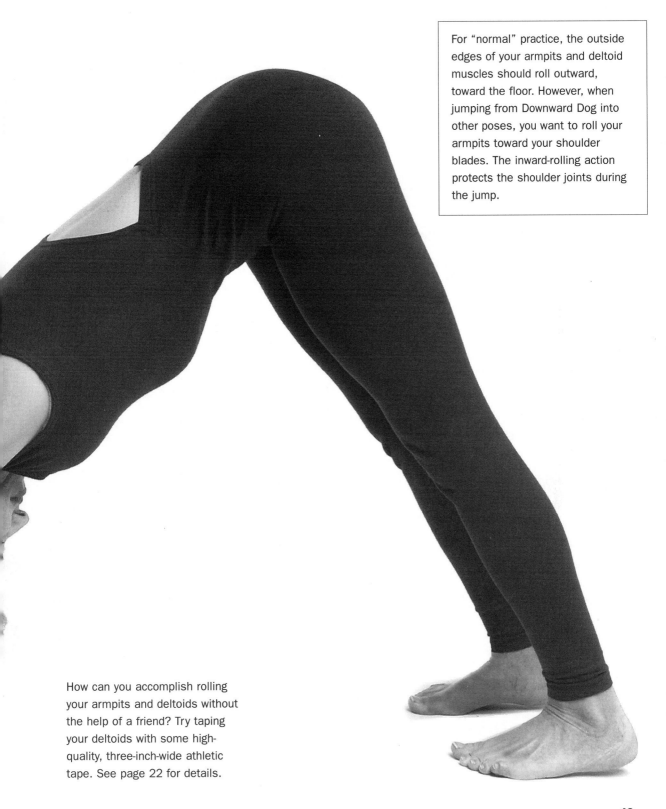

For "normal" practice, the outside edges of your armpits and deltoid muscles should roll outward, toward the floor. However, when jumping from Downward Dog into other poses, you want to roll your armpits toward your shoulder blades. The inward-rolling action protects the shoulder joints during the jump.

How can you accomplish rolling your armpits and deltoids without the help of a friend? Try taping your deltoids with some high-quality, three-inch-wide athletic tape. See page 22 for details.

Spine-Lengthening Tricks

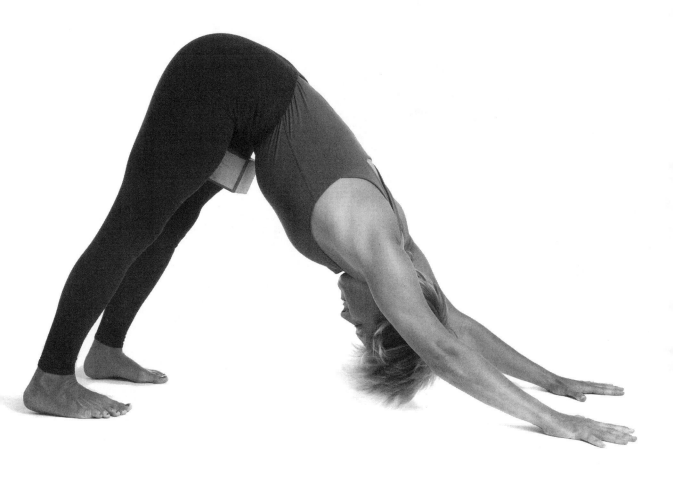

Start by kneeling on all fours. Place a block as high between your thighs as possible. Straighten your legs and come into the pose. The block automatically lifts your quads. Now, push the block behind you and feel your spine lengthen. Working on the other aspects of the pose is now much easier.

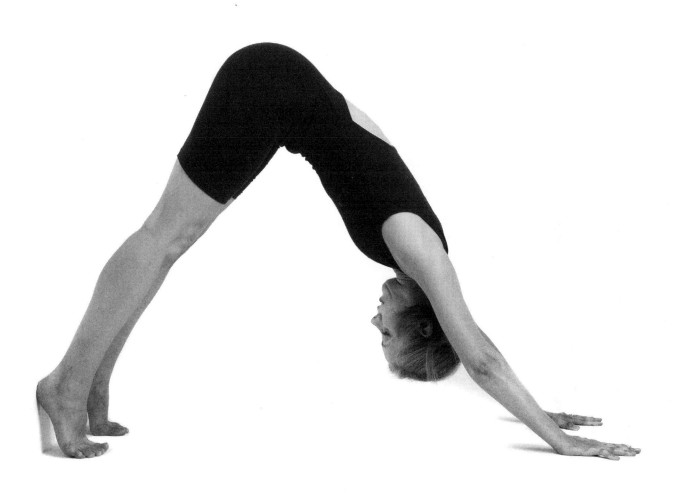

With your feet facing away from a wall, come into Dog Pose and press your heels firmly into the wall. Notice how much easier it is to press your thighs back, and in doing so, your spine lengthens and your arms and shoulders feel lighter.

Forward Forearms Trick

This trick is particularly good for those with hyperextended elbows. I have hyperextended elbows and so do most of our models—it is quite common. You can recognize hyperextension when someone's elbows are completely straight but look slightly bent or their forearms come too close to the floor in Dog Pose. For most people this is not painful, but some students simply experience elbow discomfort when performing Downward Dog or Handstand. If any of these things are true for you, try this trick.

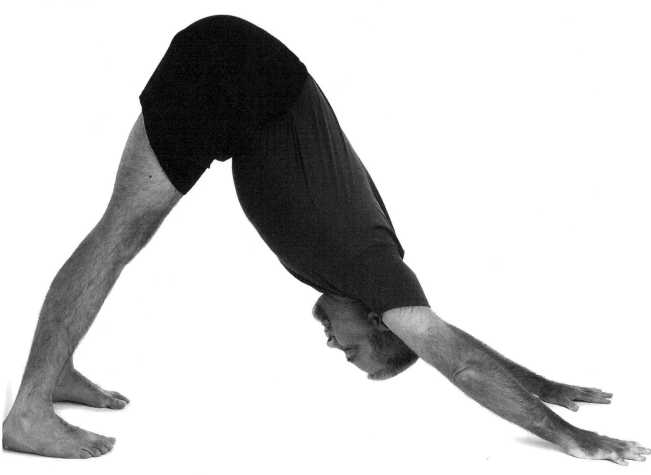

Notice Terry's forearms in this photo. His forearms and elbows are too close to the floor, putting pressure on his elbows and his shoulders.

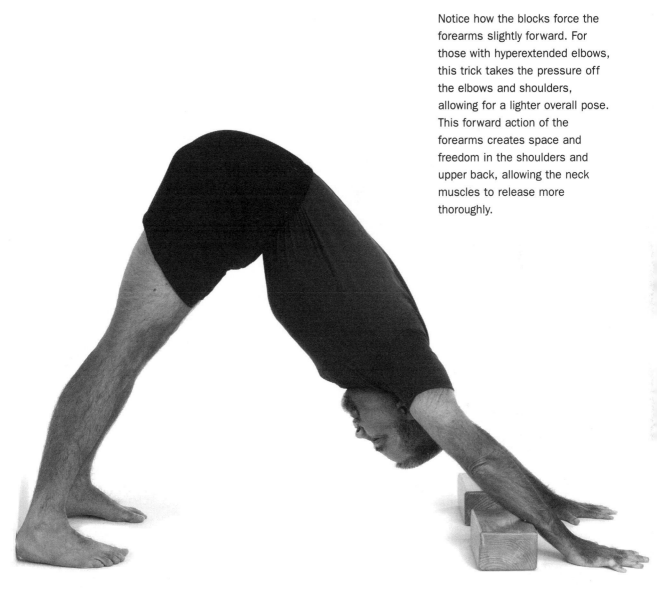

Notice how the blocks force the forearms slightly forward. For those with hyperextended elbows, this trick takes the pressure off the elbows and shoulders, allowing for a lighter overall pose. This forward action of the forearms creates space and freedom in the shoulders and upper back, allowing the neck muscles to release more thoroughly.

■ Place two yoga blocks near one end of your mat. The blocks should be shoulder-distance apart. Prepare for Dog Pose from the "all fours" position and place your hands in front of the blocks.

■ When you come up into Dog Pose, make sure that the blocks are at about the middle of your forearms.

Relief for Your Wrists

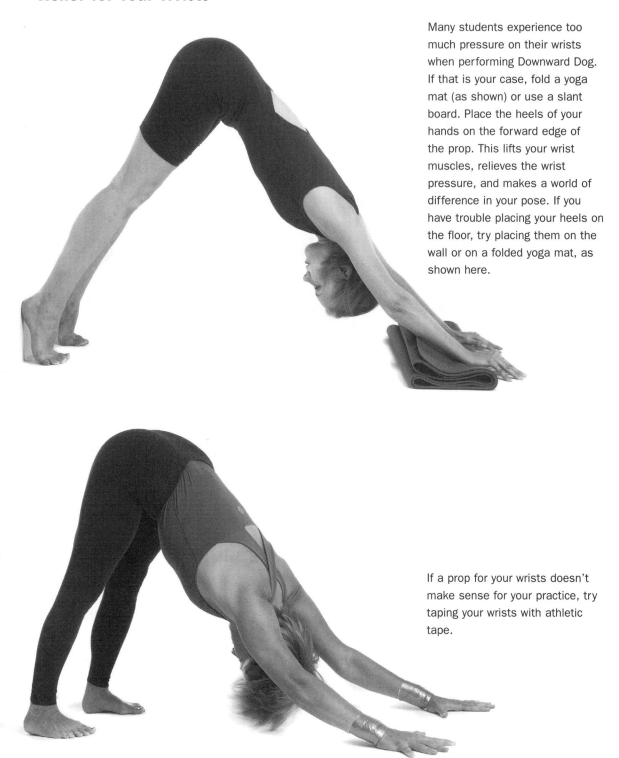

Many students experience too much pressure on their wrists when performing Downward Dog. If that is your case, fold a yoga mat (as shown) or use a slant board. Place the heels of your hands on the forward edge of the prop. This lifts your wrist muscles, relieves the wrist pressure, and makes a world of difference in your pose. If you have trouble placing your heels on the floor, try placing them on the wall or on a folded yoga mat, as shown here.

If a prop for your wrists doesn't make sense for your practice, try taping your wrists with athletic tape.

LAZY DOG TRICK

When you are too tired to practice Downward-Facing Dog, try this passive Dog Pose.

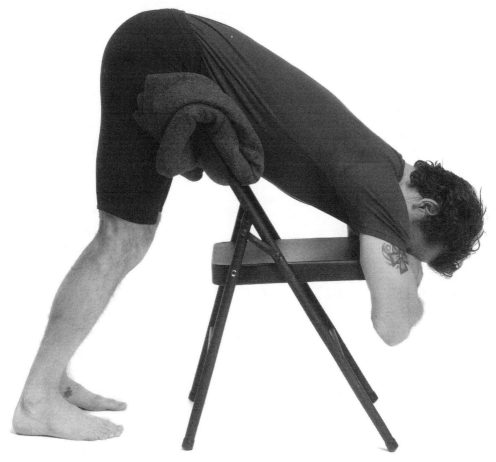

Chair-Supported Dog

This pose is comfortably done over the back of a soft, stuffed chair. But you can also use a wooden or metal chair, as shown here, by padding the top with a yoga mat, blanket, or both.

■ Place a folded yoga mat or blanket on the top of the back of the chair.

■ Lean over the chair, with the top of the chair at your hip crease.

■ Angle your torso as you would in an active Dog Pose. Hold your elbows and place your head on

your forearms so you are able to breathe and be comfortable.

■ Bend your knees if that is more relaxing.

■ Stay in this supported Dog Pose as long as you like. Notice how all of your back muscles release and soften.

Fine-Tuning

There is one excuse for not trying yoga that I hear over and over again: "I can't even touch my knees, much less my toes. How can I do yoga?"

What eludes most of these would-be yogis is that no one *is expected to be able to "do" yoga immediately. That is why it is called yoga practice. Among its many benefits, practicing yoga helps you increase your flexibility, making it possible that someday you will be able to touch your toes.*

Your Forward Bends

Touching the toes, however, is not the ultimate goal. Forward bends are much more than that. Tight hamstrings, hips, and lower backs are what usually prevent us from making contact with our toes. But more important, these constrictions often cause pain—particularly in the lower back. People often ask what causes these limitations. The answer is simple: life. We tighten up from our everyday activities—sitting or standing at our jobs, picking up our children, carrying the groceries, etc. Many of us wake up more tense than we were when we went to bed. Whatever the cause, forward bends are the prescribed antidote.

Forward bends ease the tightness in these areas. Additionally, forward bends tone the abdominal organs, lengthen and strengthen the spine and back muscles, calm the nervous system, enhance circulation, and increase overall energy.

While practicing forward bends, we feel a sense of calmness: the result of the physiological response. With a regular practice of forward bends, we begin to experience the increased energy that comes from stretching and strengthening the spine and surrounding muscles. We feel more alive, energetic, and focused. With continued practice we might just experience some benefits we never dreamed possible—like touching our toes. And after that, who knows? Just think of the possibilities!

PASCHIMOTTANASANA
Intense West Stretch

To experience the greatest benefits of this pose, it is of utmost importance to extend the spine as much as possible, and to extend it equally. This means that both sides of the torso and the front and the back of the torso must stretch evenly. This is best accomplished by grounding the hips and legs to the floor. Rolling the thighs inward and pressing the femur bones to the backs of the legs allow uniform extension of the back, enhancing both physical and spiritual equilibrium.

- Sit on the floor with your legs stretched out in front of you, feet together.

- With your hands, release your glutes outward so your sit bones are as close to the floor as possible.

- Lift your lower back and lower abdominal muscles slightly upward and inward.

- Engage your quadriceps, lifting them toward your hips.

- Press the fronts of your thighs toward the backs of your thighs, and stretch the backs of your thighs toward the floor. Make sure that the contact between the floor and the legs is maintained throughout the pose.

- Roll your thighs inward, and press the inner thighs firmly toward the floor.

- Lift your arms overhead. Bend forward from your hip crease, not from the waist.

- Extend from the base of your spine as evenly as possible and extend your sternum toward your feet.

- Place your hands around your feet or use a prop as described later.

- Continually extend your spine throughout the pose. These movements become very subtle.

- Keep your head in line with the rest of your spine. Relax your neck and shoulders.

- Do not force further extension but rather allow your body to gradually guide you.

- Stay in the position as long as you like.

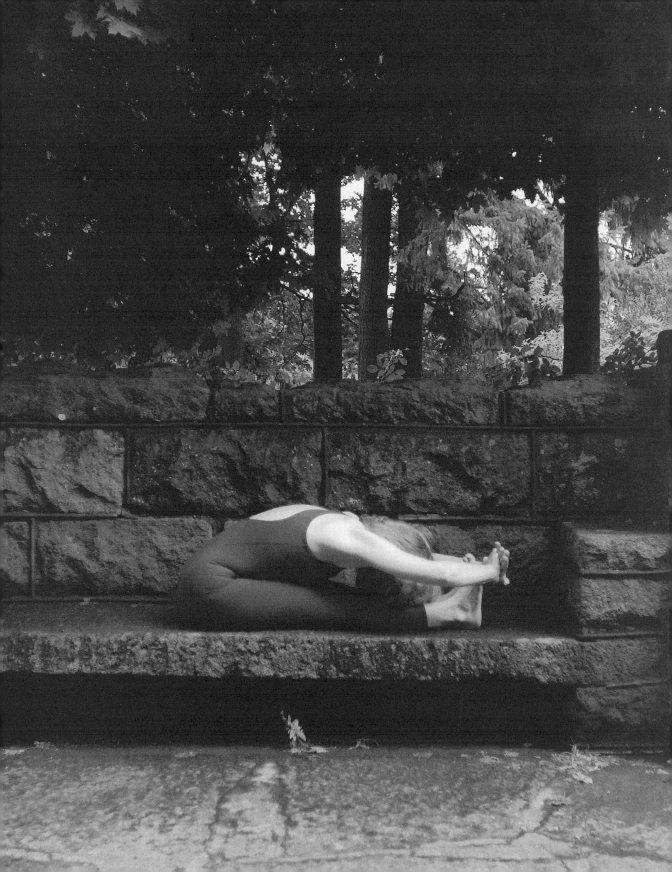

The Many Phases of Paschimottanasana

The classical version of Paschimottanasana, demonstrated on page 53, is an ideal that most of us will not realize for many decades. I say that not to discourage anyone but instead to give a realistic view of the possible. To ultimately reach that ideal and to get the most benefit for your own body, try the following tricks. They guide the body into a fuller extension of the spine and a firmer grounding of the thighs. Some of the tricks help you engage the quads and roll your thighs inward more fully. In many of these postures, you will feel more freedom and openness in your back. Beginning, intermediate, and advanced students can benefit from all of these tricks.

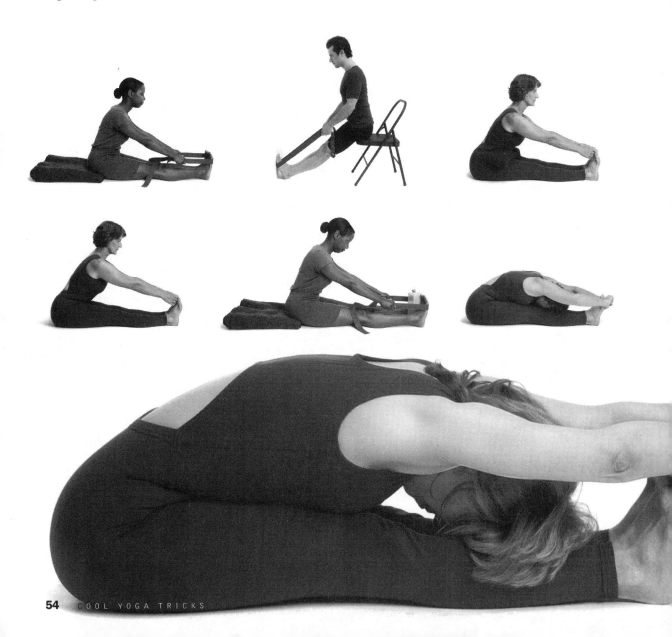

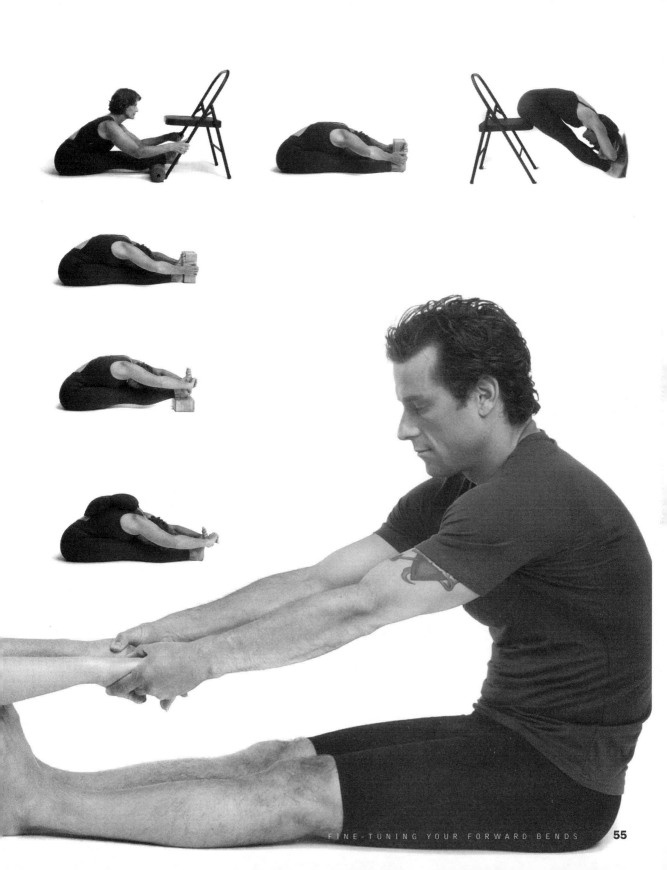

TRIANGA MUKHAIKAPADA PASCHIMOTTANASANA
Three-Footed Forward Bend

To experience the greatest benefits of this pose, it is of utmost importance to extend the spine as much as possible. This is accomplished by evenly grounding the hips and legs, including the knees, to the floor. The points of balance for this pose are the center of the extended thigh and the center of the heel.

- Sit on the floor with your legs stretched out, feet together.

- With your hands, release your glutes outward so your sit bones are as close to the floor as possible.

- Bend your left leg so that your shin is on the floor, your calf is next to your thigh, and your foot is next to your hip.

- Make sure that your thighs and knees are touching each other. Your extended-leg quadriceps should be engaged and that thigh should roll slightly in toward the floor. The bent-leg thigh and knee roll slightly outward.

- Sit equally on both hips.

- Slightly lift your lower back and abdomen up and in toward each other. Extend your spine. Lift your sternum without tightening your shoulders.

- Bring your hands overhead and, from the hip crease, bend forward and clasp your foot with your hands.

- Stretch your torso evenly, shifting your weight to the bent-leg side if you start to lose your balance.

- Extend from the base of your spine and extend your sternum toward your foot.

- Continually stretch your torso from your hip crease to your head. Be sure to stretch both sides of your waist and rib cage evenly. The movements become increasingly subtle.

- Stretch your arms from the shoulders and be sure to keep the tops of your shoulders relaxed.

- Keep your neck, throat, and face soft.

- Hold as long as you like.

- Release and switch sides.

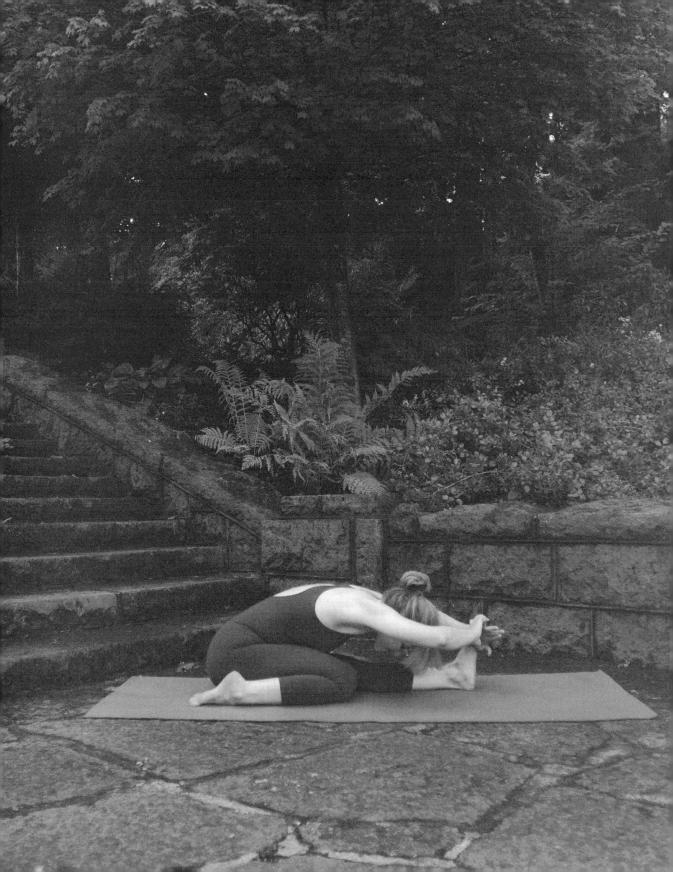

This posture can be tough even for experienced students because it requires great flexibility in the hips, knees, ankles, and feet. When many of us bring the leg back into Virasana, our lack of flexibility makes us lopsided and in danger of straining the knee. To alleviate that problem, place a folded blanket under the hip of the extended leg, then proceed into the pose. To alleviate stiffness in the ankle and feet, try the other tricks.

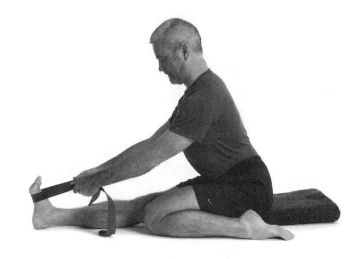

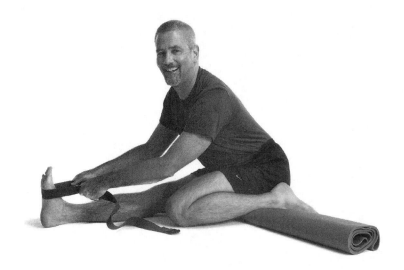

Placing a rolled blanket or yoga mat under the top of your foot helps increase flexibility in the ankle and foot. As your flexibility increases, try moving the rolled mat closer to the toes. These two poses are particularly good for runners, bicyclists, and dancers.

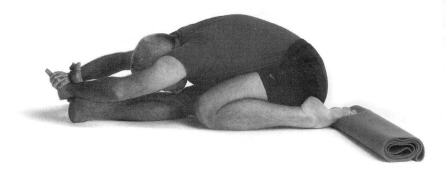

Caution: *Do not try this pose if you have to sit on more than one block when you normally practice Virasana (Hero's Pose).*

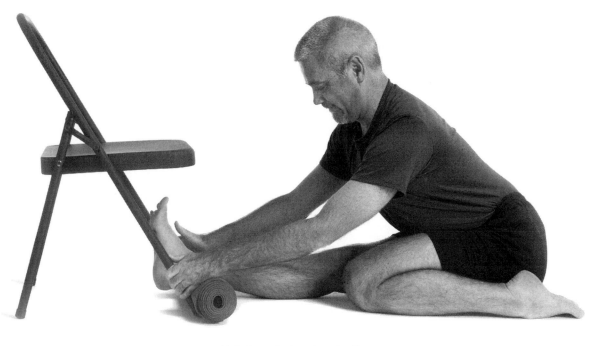

■ Using a rolled mat under the ankle and a chair to stabilize the foot helps ground the thighs properly, thus allowing more extension in the spine.

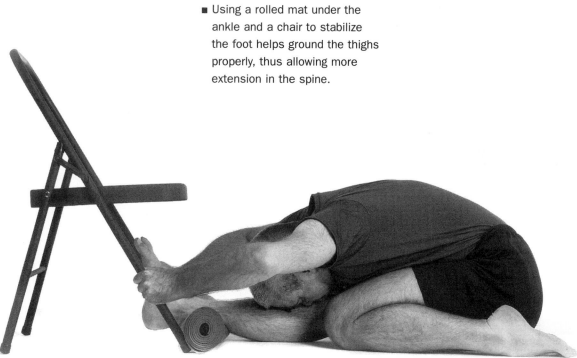

■ If you pull on the sides of the chair evenly, the two sides of your torso should stretch equally.

JANU SIRSASANA
Head-to-Knee Pose

In this pose, it is much easier to stretch the torso on the same side as the extended leg. Compensate for this tendency by maintaining a constant awareness of stretching both sides of your torso equally.

- Sit on the floor with your legs extended and your legs and feet touching.

- With your hands, release your glutes outward so your sit bones are as close to the floor as possible.

- Slightly lift your lower back and abdomen up and in toward each other. Extend your spine. Lift your sternum without lifting your shoulders.

- Bring your right hand under your right knee. Bring your leg in toward your body. Then bring the sole of your right foot to rest flat against your inner left thigh, as close to your pubic bone as possible.

- Make sure your extended leg is aligned with your hip.

- Readjust the lift of your torso.

- Engage the quadriceps of the extended leg and roll that thigh inward, pressing the inner thigh toward the floor.

- Place your right hand on the side of your left knee and slightly twist, from the bottom of your spine, toward the left. The goal is to align your spine with your extended leg.

- Maintaining the twist, lean forward from your hip crease.

- Clasp your foot with your hands.

- Keep the thigh of the extended leg firm and rolling inward.

- Extend from the base of your spine, and extend your sternum toward your foot.

- Continually stretch your torso from the hip crease to your head. Be sure to stretch both sides of the waist and rib cage evenly. The movements become increasingly more subtle.

- Relax the tops of your shoulders, your throat, your neck, and your face.

- Hold as long as you like, release, and switch sides.

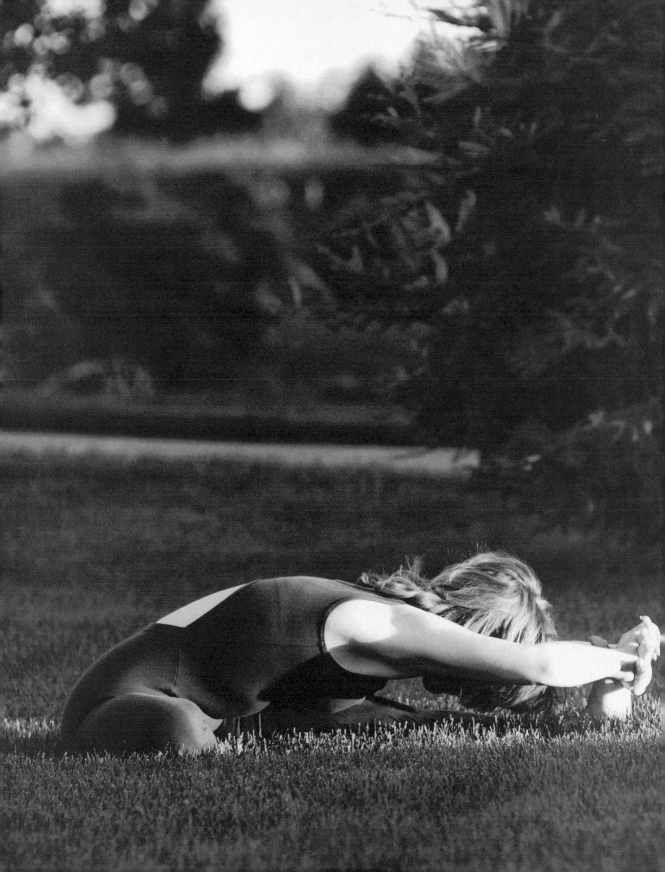

Janu Sirsasana is the classic Head-to-Knee Pose. Fortunately it can be practiced long before we can actually place our forehead on our shin. For many of us, the most difficult aspects of this pose are that the bent knee hurts and our lower backs are stiff. The following tricks can alleviate these problems.

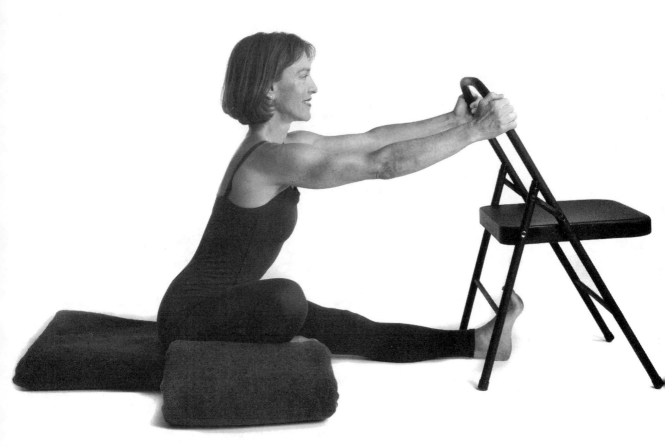

■ Place a rolled or folded blanket under the thigh of the bent leg. If you can ground this leg, the inner thigh will be able to relax more readily, which will help move your torso farther forward more evenly.

■ If your back and hamstrings are very tight, you can sit on a blanket and place your hands on the sides of a chairback or on a chair seat.

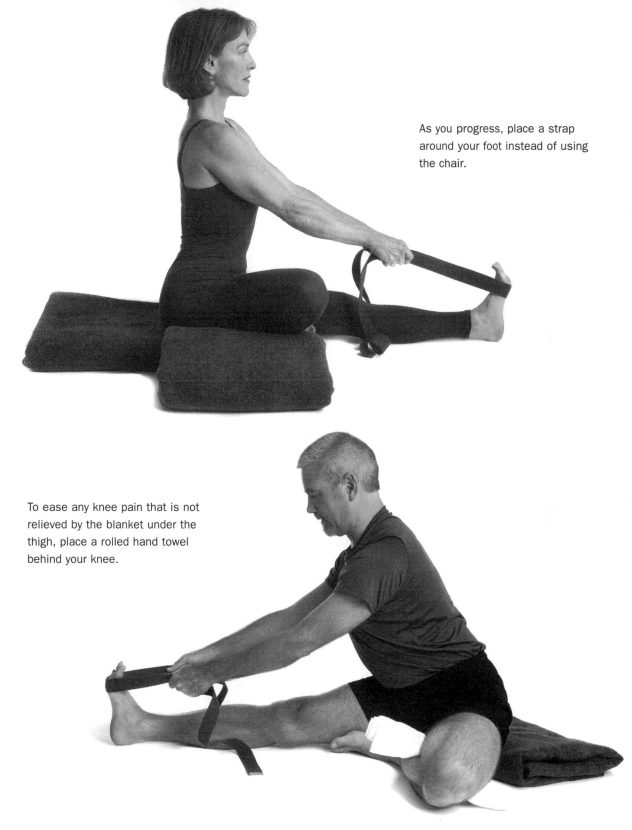

As you progress, place a strap around your foot instead of using the chair.

To ease any knee pain that is not relieved by the blanket under the thigh, place a rolled hand towel behind your knee.

UPAVISTA KONASANA
Seated Wide-Angle Pose

Upavista Konasana, Seated Wide-Angle Pose, may have the coolest name of all yoga poses. That aside, most students can perform this posture more easily than other forward bends because the hamstrings and hip flexors are not as challenged.

- Sit with your legs wide, flexing your toes toward you.

- Engage your quadriceps and roll your thighs slightly outward.

- Press the fronts of your thighs toward the backs of your thighs, and the backs of your thighs toward the floor. Make sure that the contact between the floor and your legs is maintained throughout the pose.

- Lift your lower back and abdomen and slightly bring them in toward each other.

- Lift your sternum.

- From your hip crease, lean forward, walking your fingers forward between your feet.

- Keep your lower back and abdomen moving toward each other—do not allow your lower back to collapse.

- To keep your upper back as straight as possible, extend your sternum forward.

- Continue to walk your fingers forward until the front of your torso is lying on the floor and your arms are outstretched.

- Extend the front and back of your torso evenly.

- Hold as long as you like, breathing evenly.

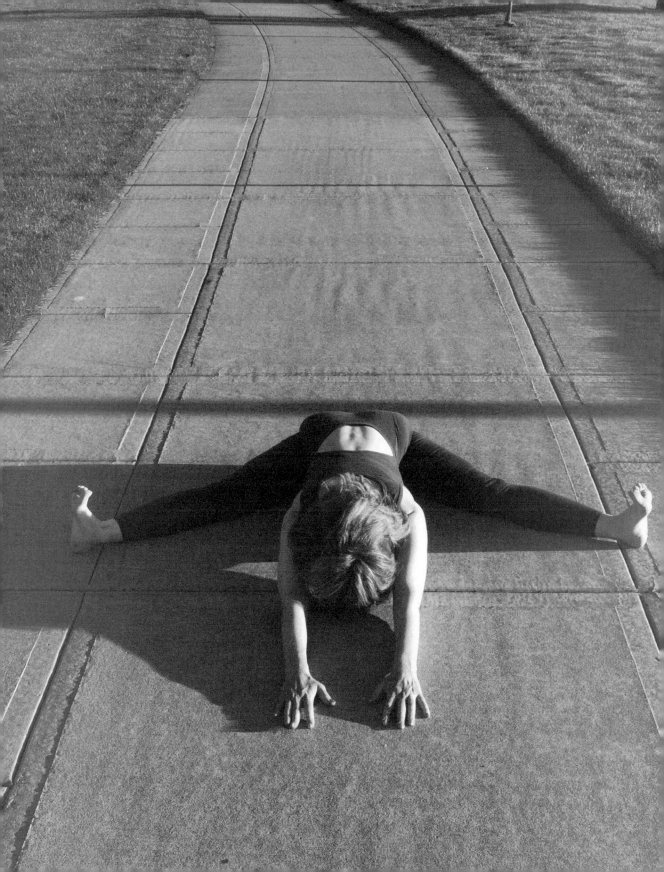

The most important aspects of Upavista Konasana are keeping the thighs firmly grounded and lengthening the spine as much as possible. And it will come as no surprise to you that the two are related. The more the thighs are grounded toward the floor, the more you will be able to extend your spine. Here are some tricks that will speed you toward placing your face on the floor. But don't be in a hurry to get there—correct posture is most important.

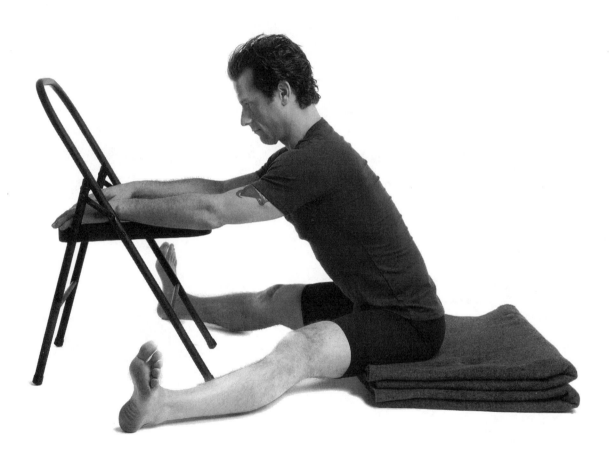

- Sit on folded blankets with your legs wide.

- Engage your quadriceps and press your thighs toward the floor.

- Have a chair or a block at its highest height in front of you.

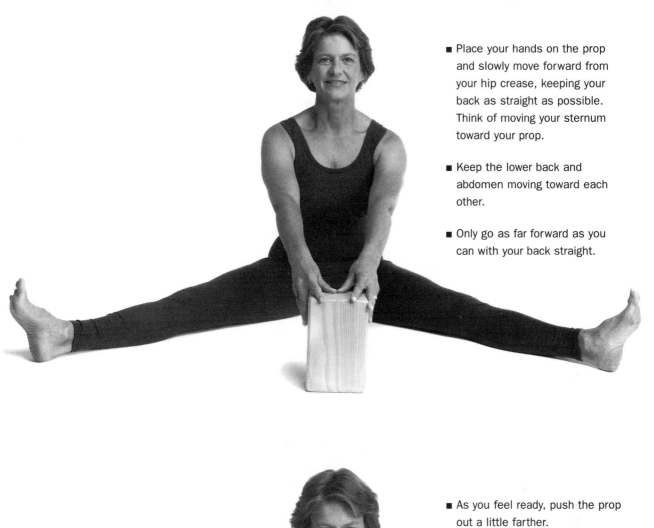

- Place your hands on the prop and slowly move forward from your hip crease, keeping your back as straight as possible. Think of moving your sternum toward your prop.

- Keep the lower back and abdomen moving toward each other.

- Only go as far forward as you can with your back straight.

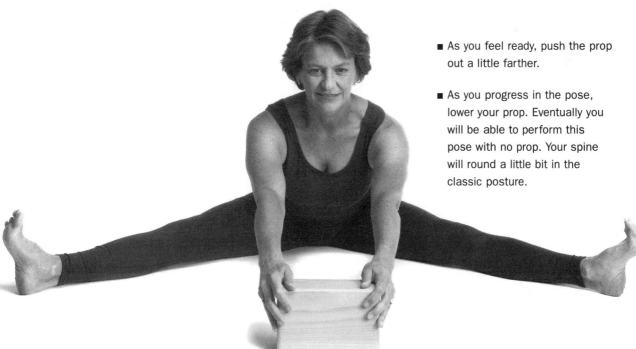

- As you feel ready, push the prop out a little farther.

- As you progress in the pose, lower your prop. Eventually you will be able to perform this pose with no prop. Your spine will round a little bit in the classic posture.

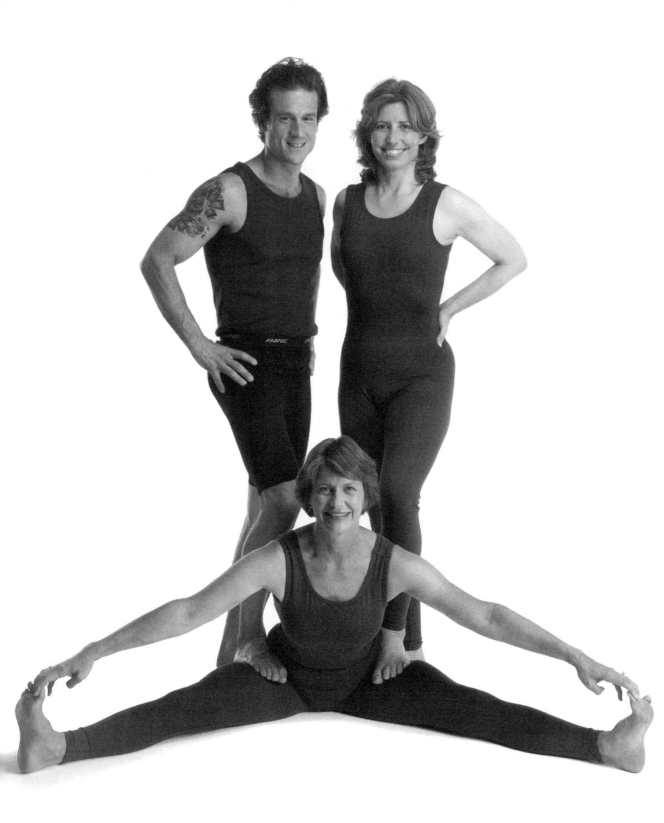

To firmly ground your thighs and enhance your ability to move forward with a straight back, have two friends stand on you. That is, each friend should place one of his feet on your thighs—approximately two inches from the hip crease. They should exert a little pressure to make sure that your thighs are as grounded as possible. Move forward into the pose as shown on the previous pages, or bring your hands to your feet. See how much farther you can advance when your friends help you.

Then try the pose without your friends' help and see how well your body's memory works. When you don't have any friends available, try this with sandbags. But they are not nearly as fun as your friends!

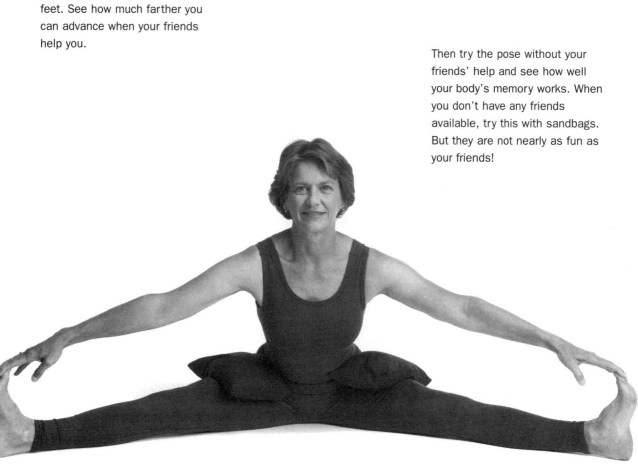

UTTANASANA
Standing Forward Bend

As in the seated forward bends, the more you can lift your thighs, roll them inward, and ground your femur bones, the more spine extension you will get in this pose.

- Stand in Samasthithi, with your feet together and making sure that your weight is evenly distributed.

- Lift your quadriceps and roll your thighs inward.

- Bring your arms overhead. Lean forward from your hip crease, bringing your head toward the floor and the front of your torso to your thighs.

- Place your hands on the sides of your feet (as shown) or hold your elbows.

- Allow your torso, neck, and head to completely release.

- Continually lift your quadriceps and roll your thighs inward.

- Spread the sit bones away from each other.

- Your hips and ankles should be aligned.

- Do not force yourself to go deeper into the pose, but rather allow your lower back, hamstrings, and the backs of your knees and calves to ease into the pose as these muscles slowly release.

- Hold as long as you like. Release by bringing your arms to the sides of your head and stand erect.

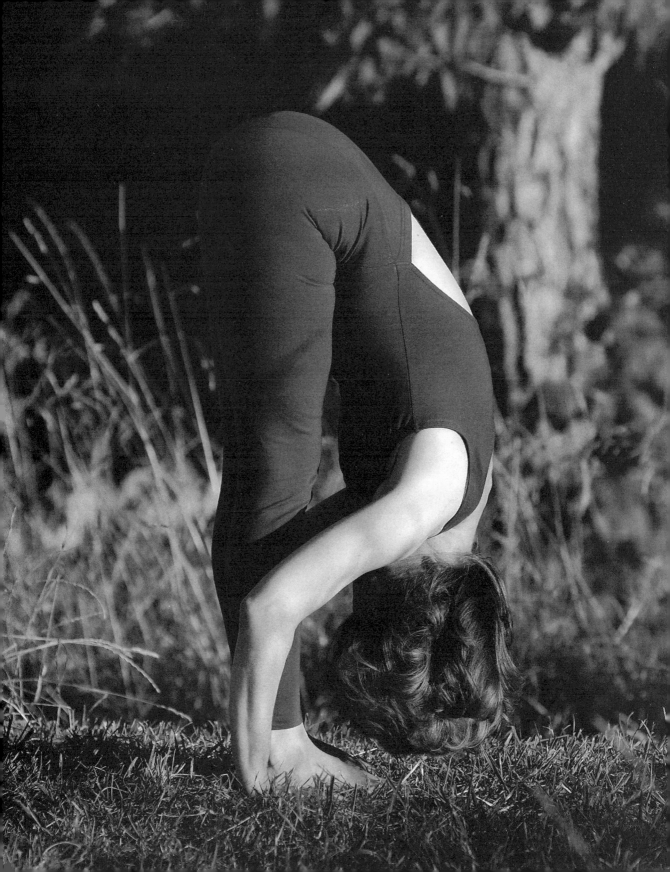

The most common complaint about Uttanasana is the pain of stretching the backs of the legs. For many people, the calves, backs of the knees, and hamstrings scream in agony. The next most common complaint is at the opposite end of the spectrum. It comes from women who are very flexible. For them, the pose is not demanding enough. The following tricks offer solutions for both types of complaints.

Tight-Hamstring Tricks

Many yoga traditions teach stiff students to bend their knees in this pose. I am of two minds about this approach. One benefit of bending the knees is that the chance of pulling a muscle is diminished. However, if the knees are bent, the tailbone can poke out, causing misalignment. If you have very tight hamstrings, try bending your knees in this pose and be aware of sensations in your lower back. Then try the following three tricks and determine which feels best for your body.

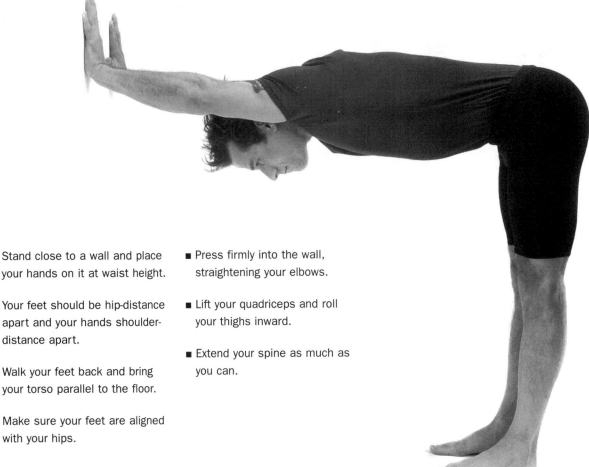

- Stand close to a wall and place your hands on it at waist height.

- Your feet should be hip-distance apart and your hands shoulder-distance apart.

- Walk your feet back and bring your torso parallel to the floor.

- Make sure your feet are aligned with your hips.

- Press firmly into the wall, straightening your elbows.

- Lift your quadriceps and roll your thighs inward.

- Extend your spine as much as you can.

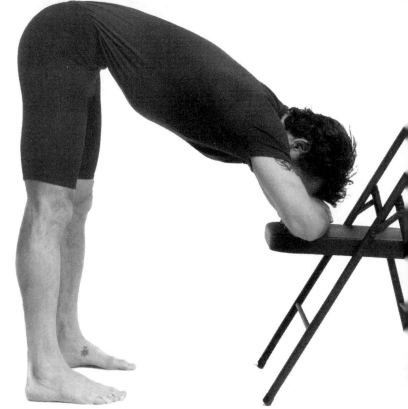

- Stand in front of a chair with your feet wider than hip distance.

- Lift your quadriceps and roll your thighs inward.

- From the hip crease, lean forward and place your hands or elbows on the chair seat.

- Allow your torso and neck to relax.

- Keep your hips and ankles aligned.

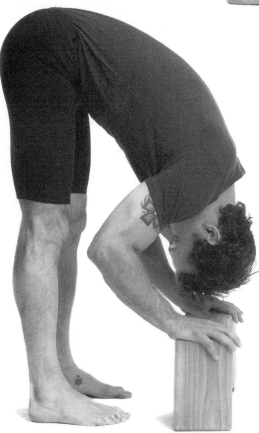

- As the backs of your legs gain flexibility, you can trade your chair for yoga blocks and narrow your stance.

Tricks for Those Who Need More Challenge in Uttanasana

- Standing, place a block between your legs as high as possible.

- Bring your feet as close together as you can.

- Come into Uttanasana, as described on page 70, and try to push the block behind you.

- Holding the block automatically lifts your quads and pushing the block behind you allows you to roll your thighs inward more easily. Both of these actions allow further extension of your spine.

- Place two yoga blocks next to each other.

- Stand on the blocks and move into Uttanasana as described on page 70.

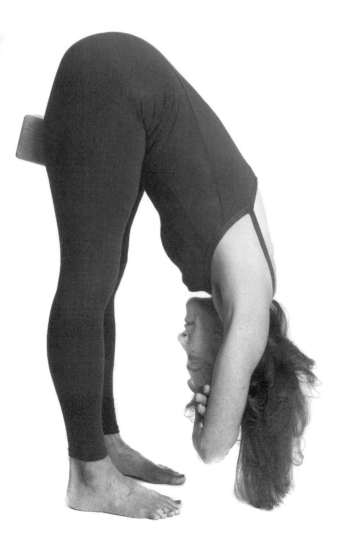

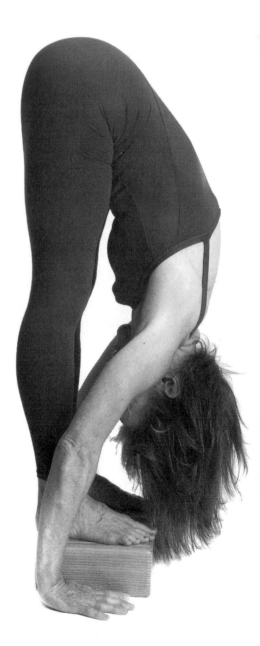

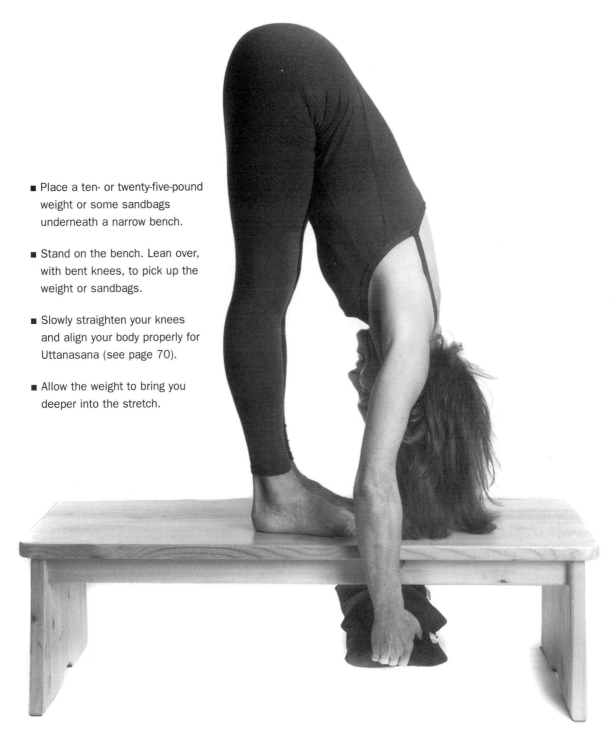

- Place a ten- or twenty-five-pound weight or some sandbags underneath a narrow bench.

- Stand on the bench. Lean over, with bent knees, to pick up the weight or sandbags.

- Slowly straighten your knees and align your body properly for Uttanasana (see page 70).

- Allow the weight to bring you deeper into the stretch.

Aligning the Hips, Feet, and Ankles in Uttanasana

Many students are unbalanced in Uttanasana, that is, their hips are behind their feet and ankles and they are counterbalancing in the pose. You can correct this tendency in three ways. 1) Keep your weight evenly distributed over your feet—front and back and side to side. 2) Rock back and forth a few times until you feel that your hips are directly above your ankles. 3) Perform the posture with your side view in a mirror. Turn your head to see if you are aligned properly and make any necessary adjustments.

BALANCED

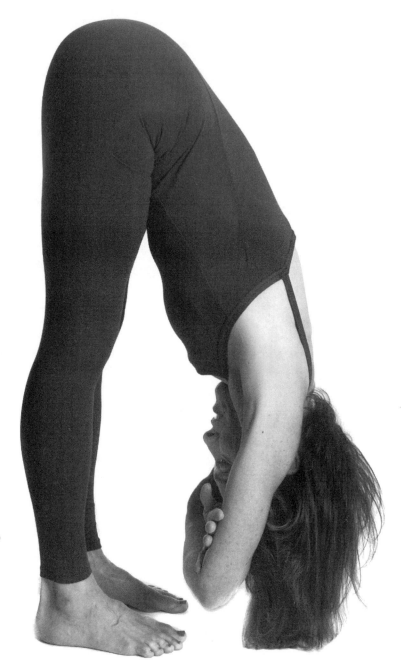

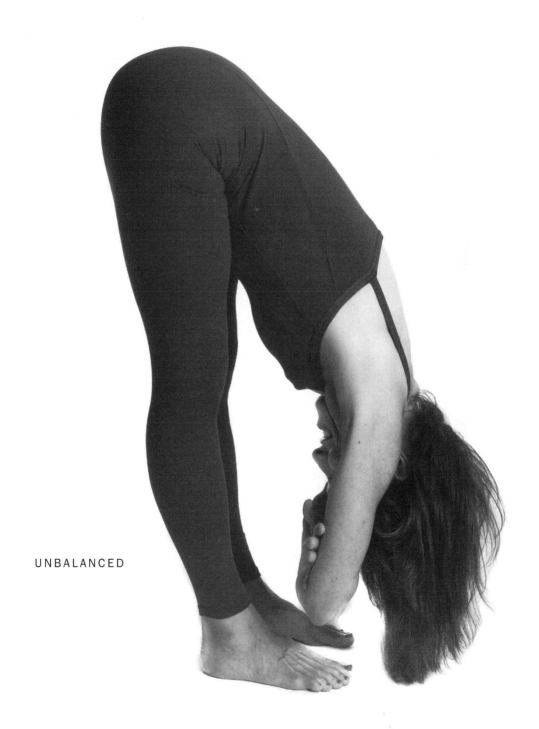

UNBALANCED

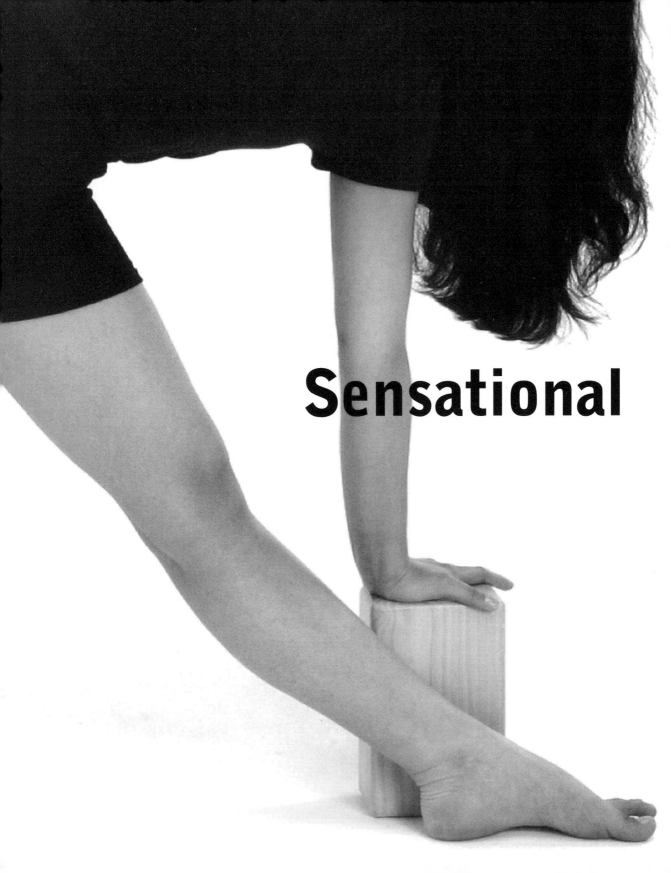

Sensational

Standing poses strengthen the body and the spirit. They invigorate us physically, mentally, and emotionally. The standing poses teach us to be simultaneously strong and flexible. Through a regular practice of standing poses, we are able to greet our daily challenges—both internal and external—with confidence, poise, balance, grace, flexibility, and concentration.

Standing Poses

The more precise our standing poses, the more energized and free we feel. Learning the specific muscular and skeletal actions in standing poses forms a foundation for back bends and inversions. In these more demanding postures, many of the same subtle movements learned in standing poses are essential to protecting ourselves from injury and to experiencing the unique benefits of back bends and inversions.

When you have a lot of time for practice, always include some standing poses. If your time is limited, standing poses are beneficial for their many empowering benefits: strength, flexibility, endurance, balance, and joy.

VRKSASANA
Tree Pose

Both physically and psychologically, Vrksasana helps us develop balance, poise, and steadiness.

- Stand with your feet together or hip-width apart. Make sure that you are aware of the four corners of your feet (see page 13).

- Lift your quads and roll your thighs inward. Lift your lower back and lower abdominal muscles and bring them slightly in toward each other. Lift your sternum and soften your shoulders, neck, and face.

- Shift your weight to your left leg and bring the sole of your right foot to the inside of your left thigh. Ideally, your heel should be at the very top of your left inner thigh, but if that is impossible for now, simply place the foot as high as you can.

- Press your foot into your thigh, and your thigh into your foot.

- Keep your right knee aligned with your hip and roll that thigh outward.

- Continually lift your left quadriceps, your lower back, lower abdomen, and sternum. Soften the tops of your shoulders.

- Bring your hands to "prayer position" at your heart, or raise your arms overhead with your arms parallel. If your arms are overhead, make sure that the elbows are straight and you are stretching your arms from the shoulders to the fingertips.

- Focus on a spot on the wall or on the floor to help you stay balanced.

- Hold the pose as long as you like and switch sides.

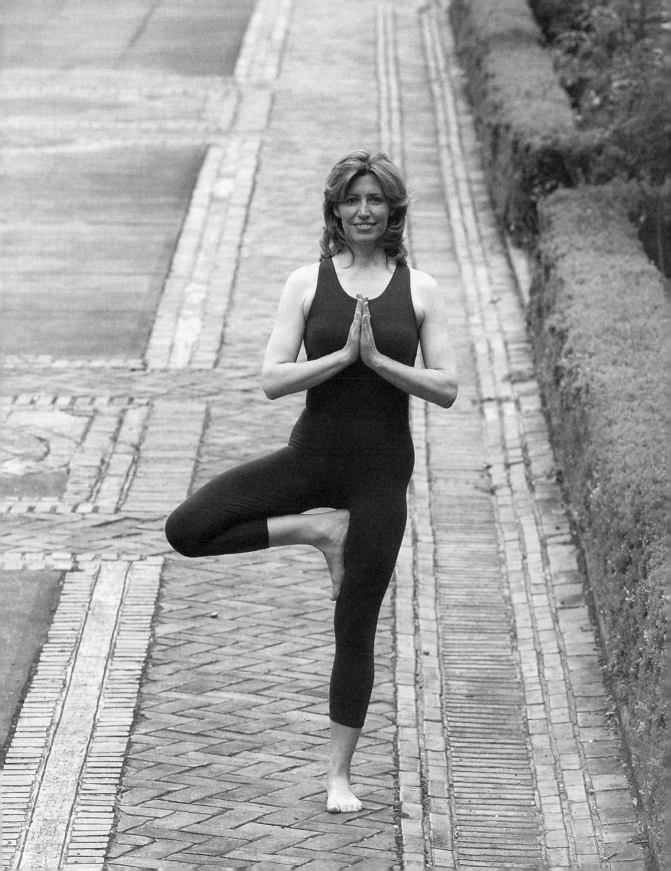

In Tree Pose, Vrksasana in Sanskrit, we balance on one leg with the sole of the opposite foot placed as high on the inside of the thigh as possible. Getting it that high—and keeping it there—can be quite tough. Additionally, the lifted leg has a tendency to angle inward, while correct alignment requires that the knee aligns with the hip. It is no surprise that both of these difficulties come from tight hips, thighs, and knees. As we practice, flexibility in these areas increases, but in the meantime try these tricks.

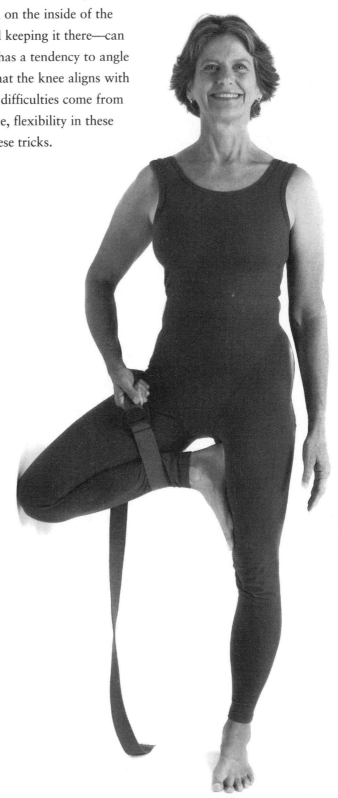

- Stand with your right side facing a wall.

- Experiment a couple of times to make sure you are at the appropriate distance by bringing the sole of your right foot to your left inner thigh. You will know that you are at the correct distance when the knee touches the wall firmly and stays put.

- From Samasthithi, shift your weight to your left leg. Bring your right knee to the wall and the sole of your right foot to the left inner thigh. Make sure your knee is aligned with your hip. Press your knee into the wall, your foot into your inner thigh, and your thigh into your foot.

- If your foot continues to slip, place a strap around the shin and hold the strap.

- Stay in the pose as long as you wish. Release and repeat on the other side.

Staying balanced in Vrksasana is also an issue for many of us. In an attempt not to fall, we often counterbalance by bringing our torso in front of our hips. Instead of counterbalancing, try the following tricks. They help with balance and with the other challenges as well.

■ Perform the posture near a wall but do not place your knee on it. Place your hand on the wall and slightly lean your torso forward. Then slightly lean backward. Find the midpoint where your torso is directly over your hips.

■ When you have found your balance, practice the pose without using the wall. But when you start to falter, place your hand on the wall to restore your balance.

Other Balancing Tricks:

1. Pick a spot on the wall or floor and concentrate on it.

2. Continually press your foot into your thigh and your thigh into your foot.

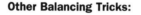

Note: If you are having trouble keeping your knee and hip aligned while practicing without the wall, grasp your thigh with your hand and roll it outward. Be near a wall or have a chair handy, just in case.

UTTHITA TRIKONASANA
Extended Triangle Pose

There are many variations of Utthita Trikonasana—Extended Triangle Pose—taught by the different yoga traditions. In some versions of Trikonasana the feet are fairly close together. In this version the feet are wide apart, allowing for a fuller extension of the spine. This creates more space between the vertebrae and more ease of movement. If you are accustomed to a narrower stance in your Triangle Pose than the stance recommended here, I ask that you try this version a few times and see if it gives you more freedom of movement and more energy. If it doesn't, do the version that is right for your body.

- Stand with your feet four to four and a half feet apart. Adjust the width of your feet according to your height.

- Turn your right foot out to ninety degrees and your left foot slightly in, about ten to fifteen degrees.

- Align the heel of your right foot with the arch of your left foot. Make sure that you are pressing the four corners of your feet into the floor. (See page 13.)

- Lift your quadriceps and roll your thighs outward—and keep them lifted and rolled throughout the entire pose.

- Press your forward hip deep into your body and keep it moving inward throughout the posture.

- Lift your lower back and your lower abdominal muscles.

- Extend your arms fully, aligning your hands with your shoulders. Relax the tops of your shoulders.

- Shift your hips toward the left.

- From the hip crease, laterally move your torso toward the right, extending the underside of your torso as much as you extend the upper side of your torso.

- Place your right hand on the floor, your shin, or your ankle.

- Rotate your torso slightly backward so your torso and hips are aligned.

- Press the fronts of your thighs toward the backs of your thighs.

- Press the inner thighs toward the outer thighs.

- Bring your left arm overhead, keeping it aligned with your shoulder. Stretch your left arm upward and press your right hand firmly into the floor, leg, or prop, which makes more space between your shoulder blades.

- Gently turn your head to gaze at your upper hand.

- While you are in the pose, continue to make the subtle adjustments that are recommended above.

- Hold as long as you like. Release and repeat on the other side.

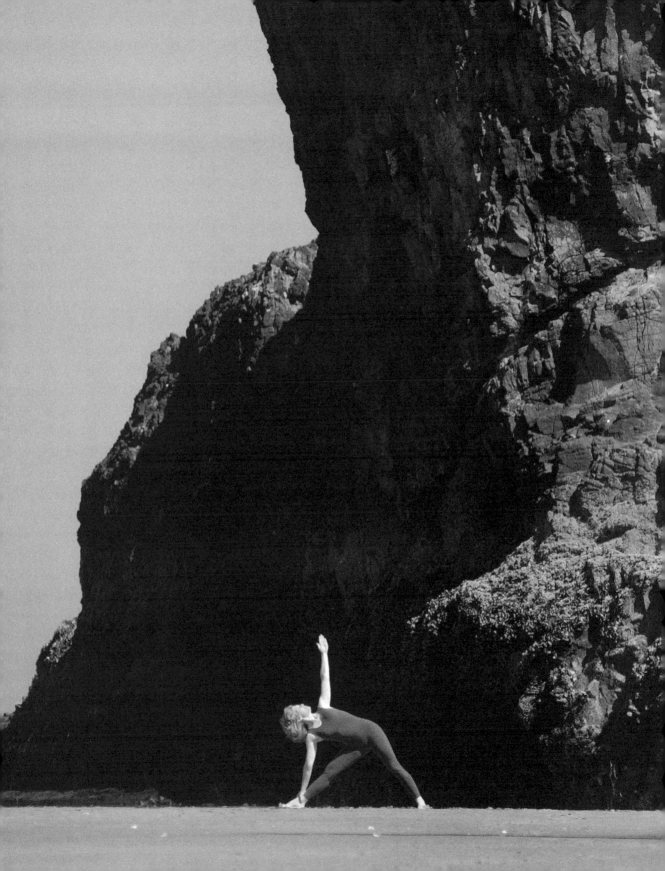

As in all yoga poses, there are many subtleties to Trikonasana—lifting and rolling the thighs outward, full extension of the spine, moving into the pose from the hip crease, aligning the torso with the hips, and rotating the head. Practice some of the thigh-lifting and -rolling tricks demonstrated in "Getting Started" (pages 10–27). From there, we will dissect Trikonasana and its accompanying challenges with the following tricks.

Thigh-Rolling Tricks

Keeping the back thigh outwardly rotated can be accomplished more easily if you place the side of your back foot against a wall. Press the edge of the foot firmly into the wall and feel the difference in your thigh.

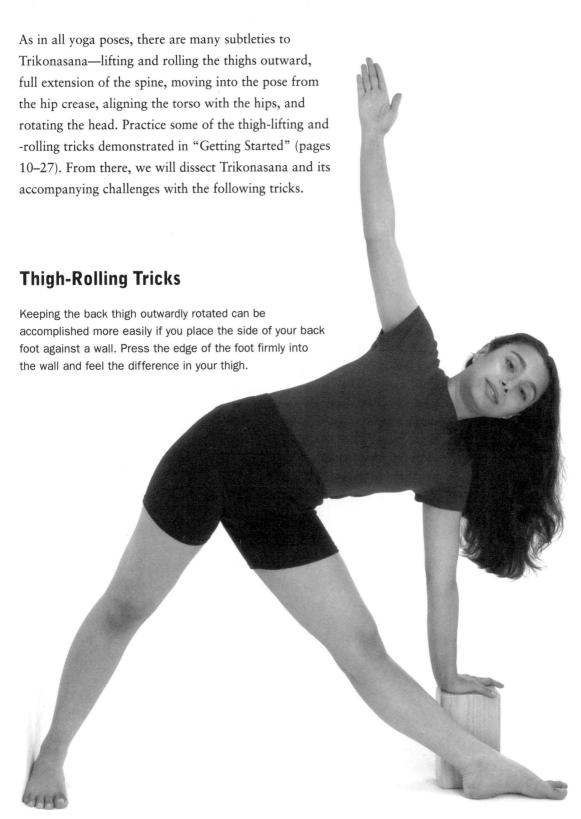

Assume the pose and have a friend help you outwardly rotate your thighs throughout your pose. See if you can maintain that rotation when he lets go. When you are alone, roll your thighs outward with your hands prior to coming into the pose. (See page 18.)

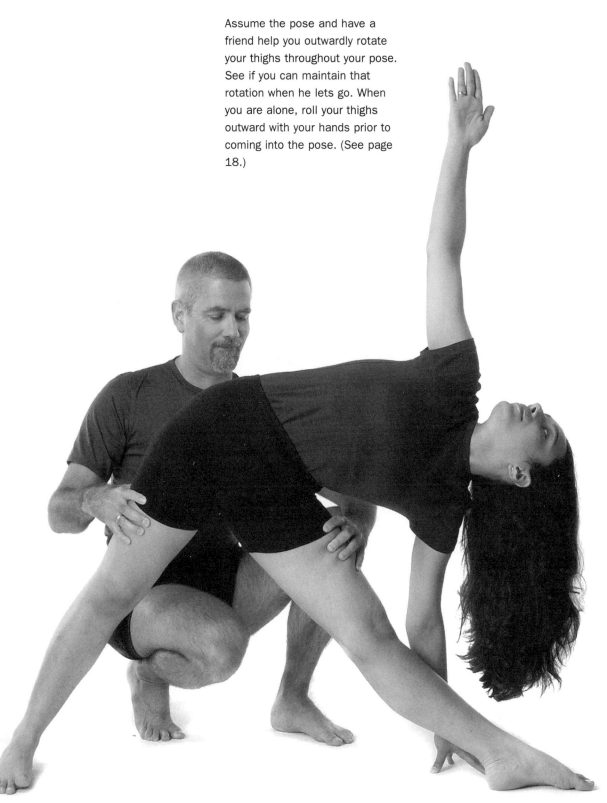

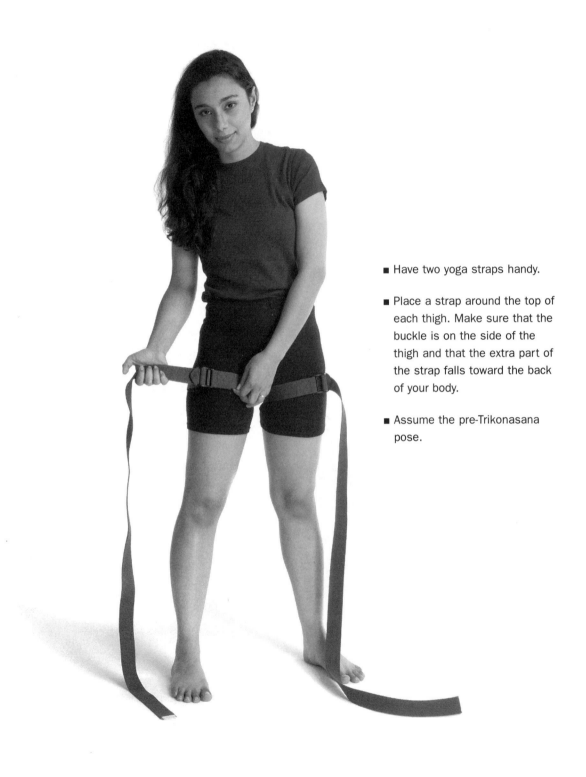

- Have two yoga straps handy.

- Place a strap around the top of each thigh. Make sure that the buckle is on the side of the thigh and that the extra part of the strap falls toward the back of your body.

- Assume the pre-Trikonasana pose.

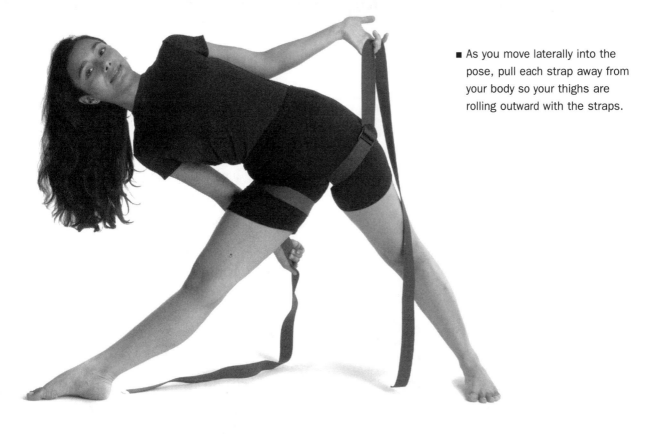

- As you move laterally into the pose, pull each strap away from your body so your thighs are rolling outward with the straps.

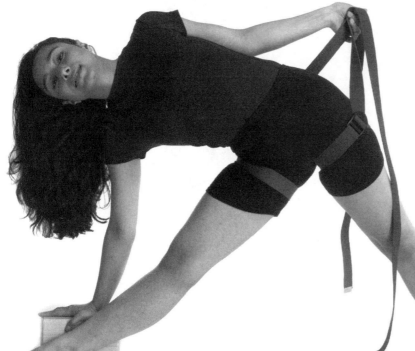

- Transfer your right strap into your left hand as you place your right hand on the block.

- As you are in the pose, pull both straps behind you to continue the outward rolling action.

- Stay in the pose as long as you like. As you release, continue to pull the straps backward.

- Release the straps and practice this trick on your left side.

Extending the Torso Evenly

Many of us want to advance in a pose more quickly than our bodies want to proceed. For example, in Trikonasana many students place their hand on their ankle or on the floor before their bodies are ready for such an action. At its worst, this eagerness can damage the spine by creating a gross misalignment. It is best to use the following tricks to practice fully extending the spine. You will be amazed at how much more energy and freedom you will experience when you do a version of Trikonasana that is right for your body.

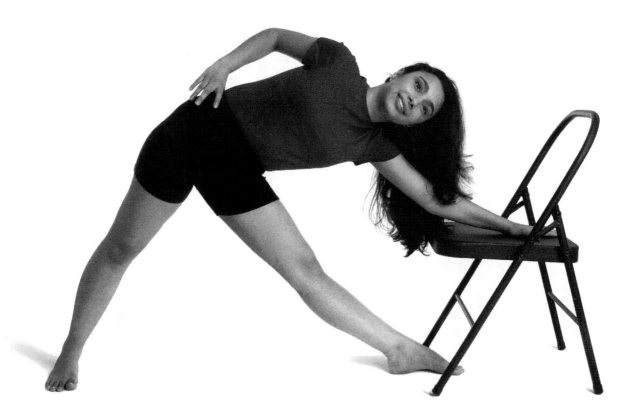

- Come into Trikonasana as you normally would.

- Depending on your freedom of movement in this pose, place your hand on a chair seat or a block.

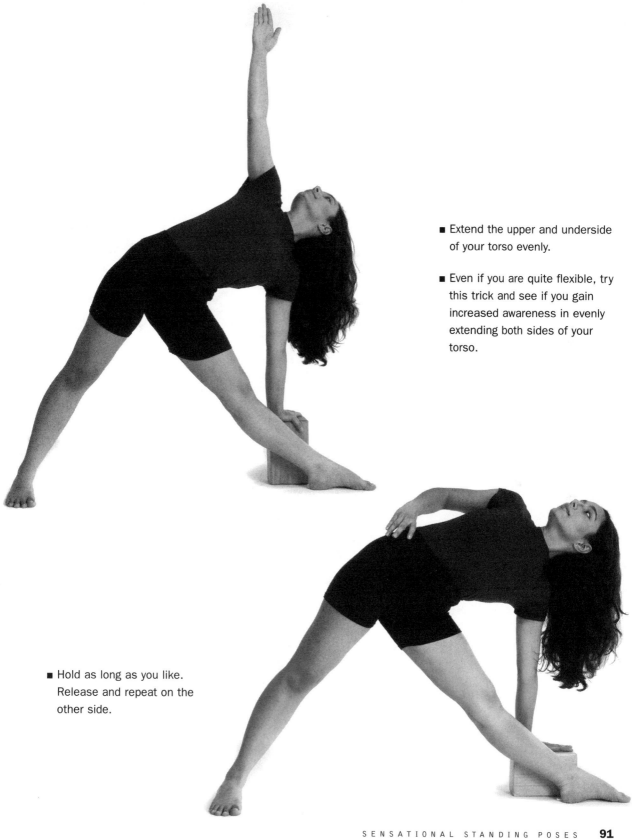

- Extend the upper and underside of your torso evenly.

- Even if you are quite flexible, try this trick and see if you gain increased awareness in evenly extending both sides of your torso.

- Hold as long as you like. Release and repeat on the other side.

Moving from the Hip Crease

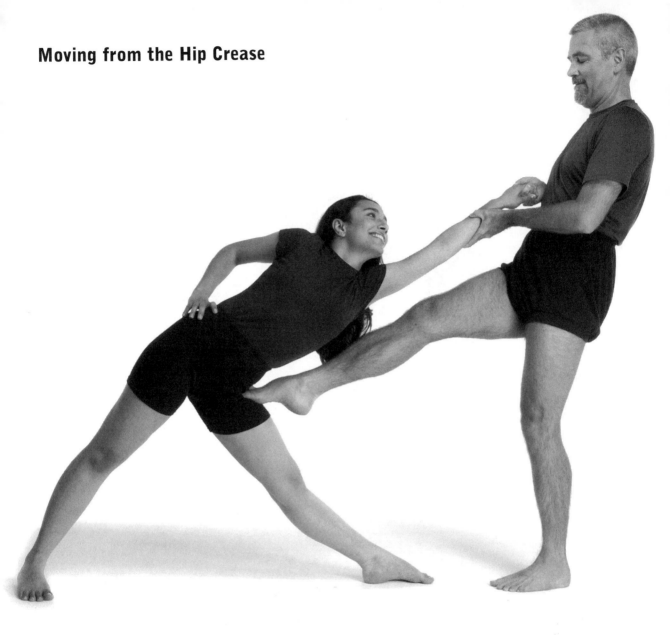

One way to learn the action of moving from the hip crease is to have a friend place his foot in your hip crease and pull you forward as you move into Trikonasana. Have your friend really pull you out, extending your spine as much as possible before he helps you place your hand on your ankle or prop.

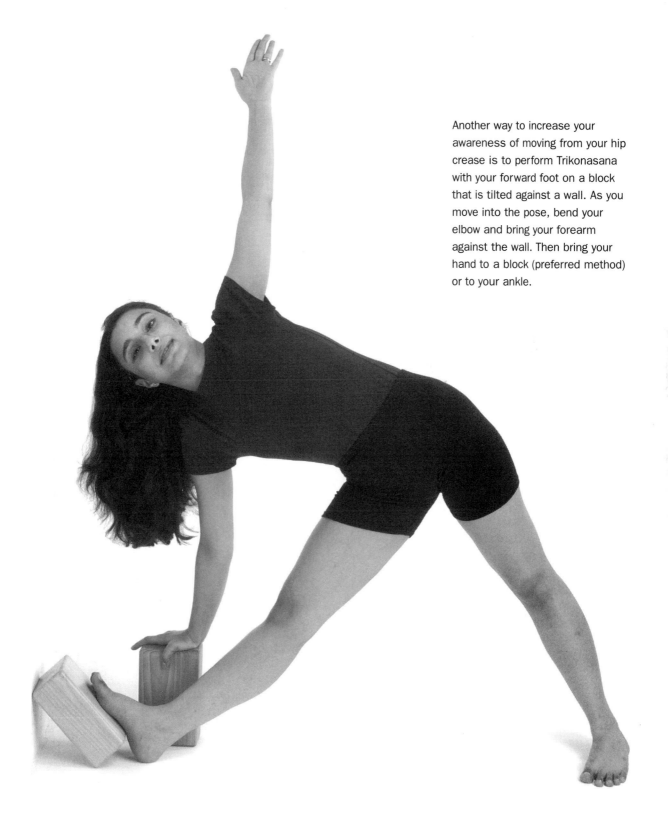

Another way to increase your awareness of moving from your hip crease is to perform Trikonasana with your forward foot on a block that is tilted against a wall. As you move into the pose, bend your elbow and bring your forearm against the wall. Then bring your hand to a block (preferred method) or to your ankle.

VIRABHADRASANA II
Warrior II

When doing Virabhadrasana II, many students feel as though their body is being split in half. This feeling comes from a full expansion of both sides of the body. We feel that split-in-half feeling the most when our inner thighs and hips are tight. Performed as well as possible, this pose will help release that tightness and will build leg, lower back, and abdominal strength.

- Stand with your feet four to four and a half feet apart and your arms extended out at shoulder level. Adjust the distance between your feet for your height. You will know that your feet are too wide if, when you are fully in the pose, your calf and thigh form an obtuse angle. Your feet are too close together if your calf and thigh form an acute angle.

- Turn the right foot out to ninety degrees and the left foot slightly in. Align the heel of the forward foot with the arch of the back foot.

- Make sure that you are aware of the four corners of your feet. (See page 13.)

- Lift your quadriceps and roll your thighs outward.

- Lift your lower back and lower abdomen and move them slightly in toward each other.

- Lift your sternum but keep the tops and backs of the shoulders relaxed.

- Press your forward hip deep into your body and keep it moving inward throughout the pose.

- Bend your forward knee into a right angle.

- Keep the back foot firmly pressing into the floor.

- Continually lift your lower back, lower abdomen, and sternum.

- Keep your torso directly over your hips and facing forward. Make sure that your torso does not tilt to the left or right or lean forward or backward.

- Back-leg instructions: Press the front of the thigh toward the back of the thigh, and press the inner thigh toward the outer thigh.

- Continually rotate both thighs outward.

- Lift your torso so much that you feel as though you will lift it off your hips (or imagine that you are lifting your torso that much).

- Slowly turn your head toward the forward hand and gaze out over your hand.

- Hold as long as you like. Release and repeat on the other side.

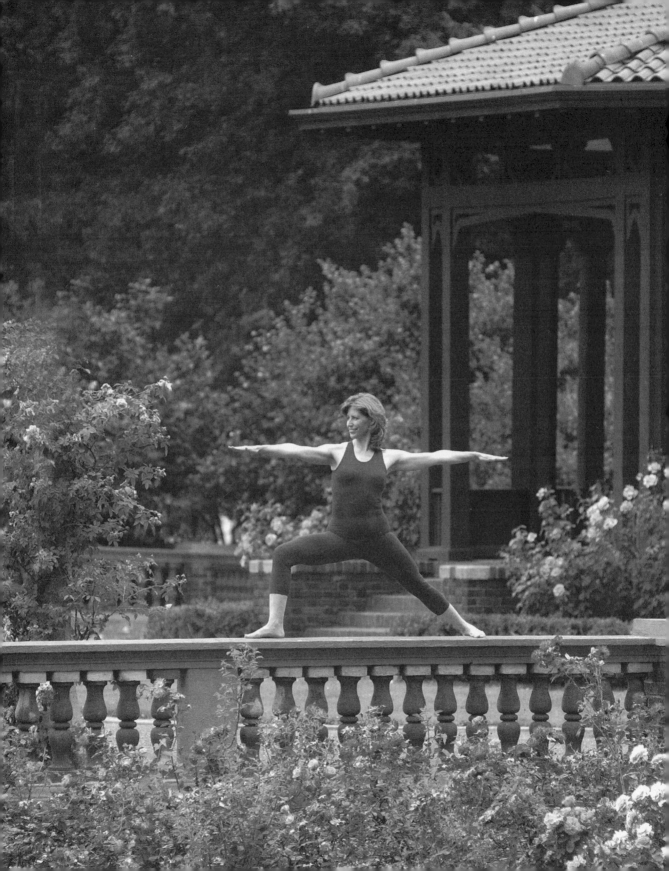

For most students, Virabhadrasana II is the easiest of the primary standing poses. Nonetheless there are challenges. For example, for many beginners the knee and the hip will not align. This is primarily due to tight inner thighs and outer hips. Beginners, then, should practice this pose without bending the forward leg into a right angle, which is safer because it puts less strain on the knee. The right angle will come naturally as your flexibility increases.

Another challenge for many students is keeping their torso directly over their hips. Many beginning students lean their torso forward of the hips or toward the front leg. Also common is "resting" in the lower back rather than lifting the lower back muscles. It is absolutely necessary to lift the lower back muscles. In daily life, "Resting" in our lower back often leads to spinal problems. By lifting the lower back and lower abdominal muscles, we strengthen these muscles, thereby helping to prevent or eliminate back pain. Try these tricks to help you overcome both of these challenges.

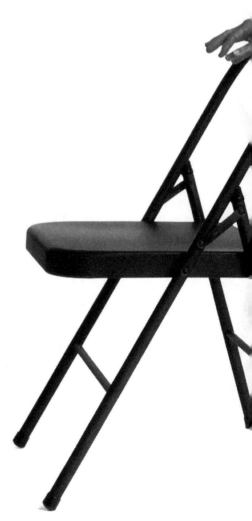

- Place a chair in front of your mat, with its back facing you, before practicing the pose.

- Assume the starting position for Warrior II.

- Place your hands on the top of the chair. Come into the pose (as otherwise described on page 94). Once your knee is bent, move the chair so it is centered in front of your hips.

- If your chair is directly in front of your hips and your torso is in front of the chair, then you are correctly aligned right to left. If not, adjust your torso.

- Press your palms or heels of your hands firmly down on the chair and, with that leverage, lift and lengthen your spine and your lower back and abdominal muscles.

- With your hands on the chair, slowly lean your torso in front of your hips. Then slightly move your torso backward. With your awareness, find the midpoint where your torso and hips are aligned.

- Consciously lift your spine, lower back, and abdominal muscles, again using the leverage of the chair to help you.

- Stay in the posture as long as you like. Release and repeat on the other side.

- Practice often to help increase your lower back strength and awareness more quickly. Alternate this trick with practicing without the chair to determine your progress.

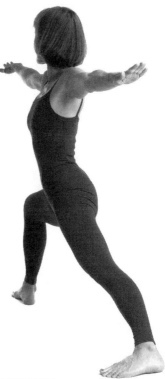

INCORRECT
ALIGNMENT

Note that in the incorrect alignment photo Julie's torso is forward of her hips and she is leaning toward her forward leg. Julie naturally has a sway back, as many people do. Julie says that through her yoga practice, and specifically by lifting her spine and lower back and abdominal muscles in her standing poses, she has strengthened her back and has greatly reduced the associated lower back pain.

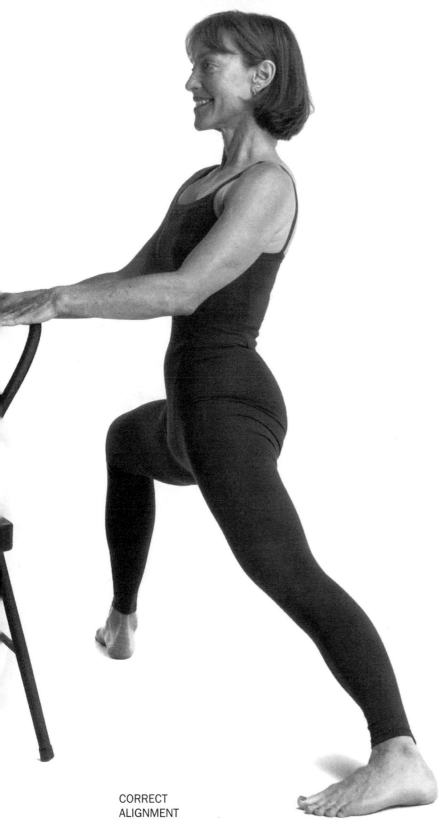

CORRECT
ALIGNMENT

Increasing Inner Thigh Flexibility

This trick will enhance your ability to keep your knee and hip aligned when you assume a right angle with your forward leg. It also helps you get the feeling of the full Warrior II extension—that split-in-half sensation. Try this trick with a friend and then be your friend's assistant.

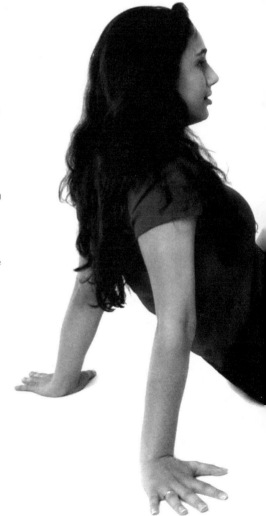

- Assume the starting position for Warrior II, with your back heel and hips against a wall. Make sure that your front heel and back arch are aligned.

- Come into the pose with your friend sitting in front of you.

- Have your friend place her feet on your inner thighs and roll your thighs outward (toward the wall). It is difficult not to laugh throughout this trick.

- Be sure to maintain all of the alignment instructions found on page 94.

- Hold the pose as long as you like. Release and repeat on the other side.

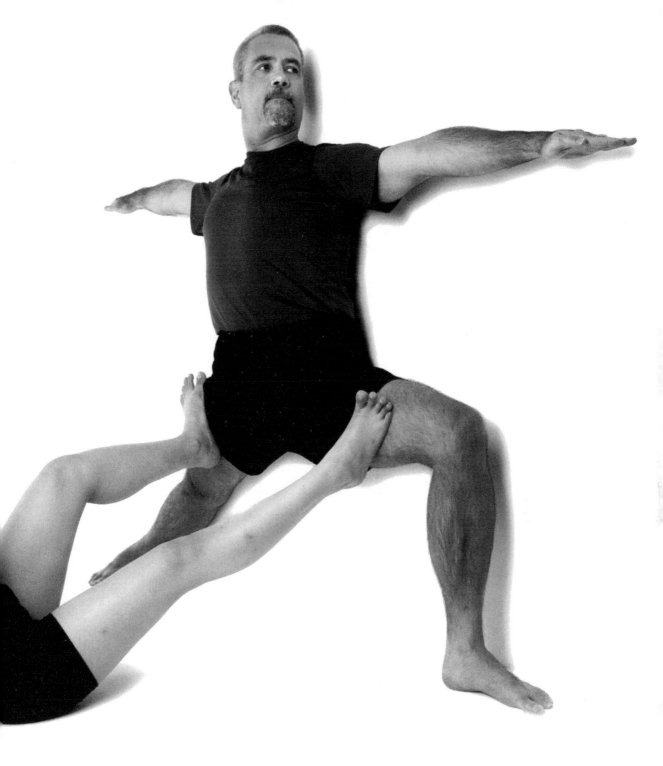

More Thigh-Rolling Tricks

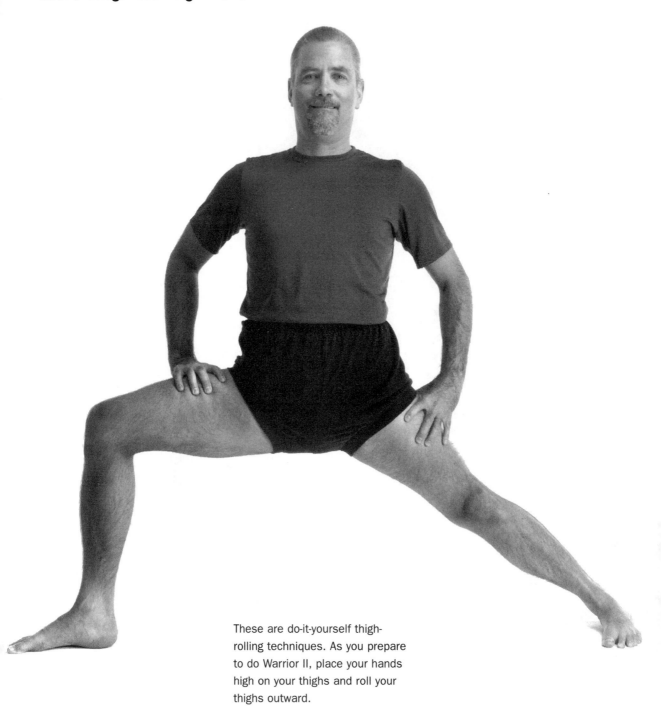

These are do-it-yourself thigh-rolling techniques. As you prepare to do Warrior II, place your hands high on your thighs and roll your thighs outward.

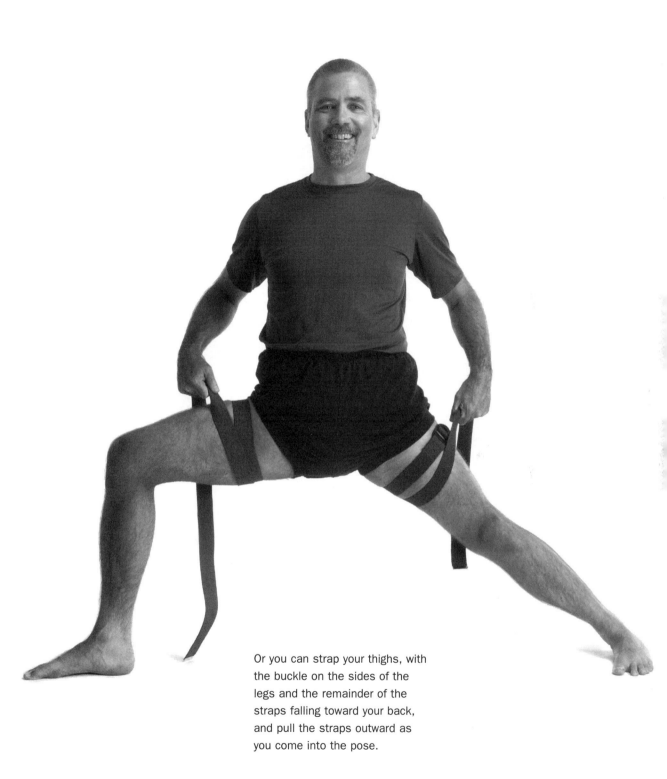

Or you can strap your thighs, with the buckle on the sides of the legs and the remainder of the straps falling toward your back, and pull the straps outward as you come into the pose.

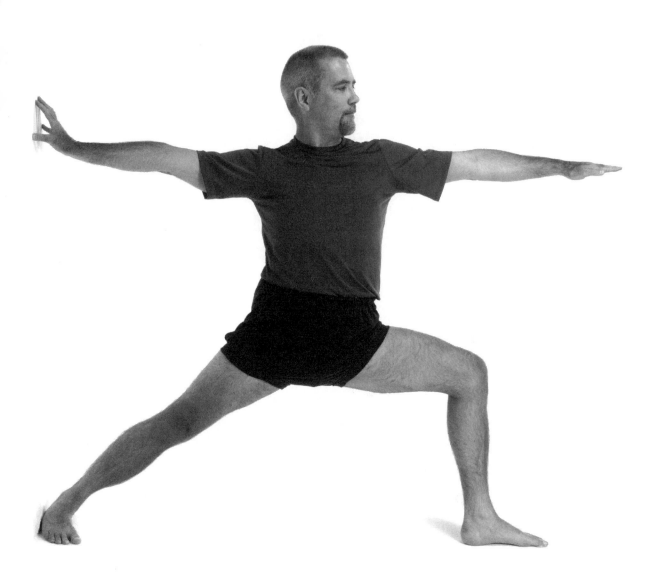

Don't forget to practice the pose
with your back foot pressing into
the wall. It helps to roll your back
thigh outward. If you keep your
hand on the wall, it helps you
keep your torso centered over
your hips.

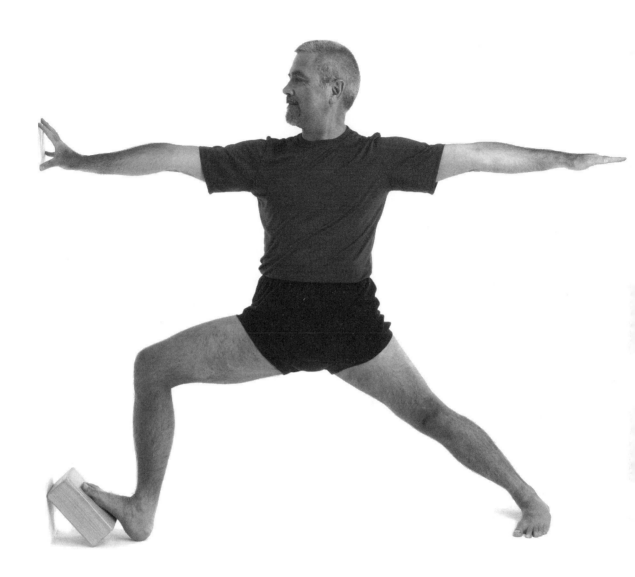

You can also practice Warrior II with your forward foot on a block. This trick has many benefits: It fosters bringing your forward hip deep into your body; it takes pressure off your knee and builds strength in the quadriceps, and it helps lift your lower back.

UTTHITA PARSVAKONASANA
Extended Side-Angle Pose

In Utthita Parsvakonasana, Extended Side-Angle Pose, the side of the torso stretches intensely over your thigh, which is parallel to the floor. Your thigh and calf form a right angle and you strongly stretch your arm past your head.

- Stand with your feet four to four and a half feet apart.

- Turn your left foot out ninety degrees and your right foot in about fifteen degrees. Make sure that you are aware of the four corners of your feet. (See page 13.)

- Extend your arms so that they are shoulder height and stretch evenly from your shoulders to your fingertips.

- Engage your quadriceps and rotate your thighs outward. Maintain this action throughout the posture.

- Lift your lower back and lower abdominal muscles and move them in toward each other slightly. Lift your sternum and keep the tops of your shoulders relaxed.

- Press your forward hip deep into your body and keep it moving inward throughout the posture.

- Relax the tops of your shoulders, your neck, your throat, and your face.

- Bend your forward leg into a right angle, as in Virabhadrasana II.

- Keeping your torso facing your front, from the hip crease laterally move the right side of your torso over your leg.

- Bring your left hand to the floor on the outside of your foot (or bring your hand to a prop as described on page 106). Bring your right arm over your head, with your palm facing the floor and your upper arm over your ear.

- Stretch from the outer edge of your back heel to your fingertips.

- Slowly turn your head to gaze at your arm.

- Press the bent thigh into your arm and your arm into the thigh.

- Rotate your torso slightly backward so that it will be aligned with your legs and hips.

- Extend the underside of your torso as much as you can.

- Hold the posture as long as you like.

- To release, come back into Virabhadrasana II. Release that pose and repeat on the other side.

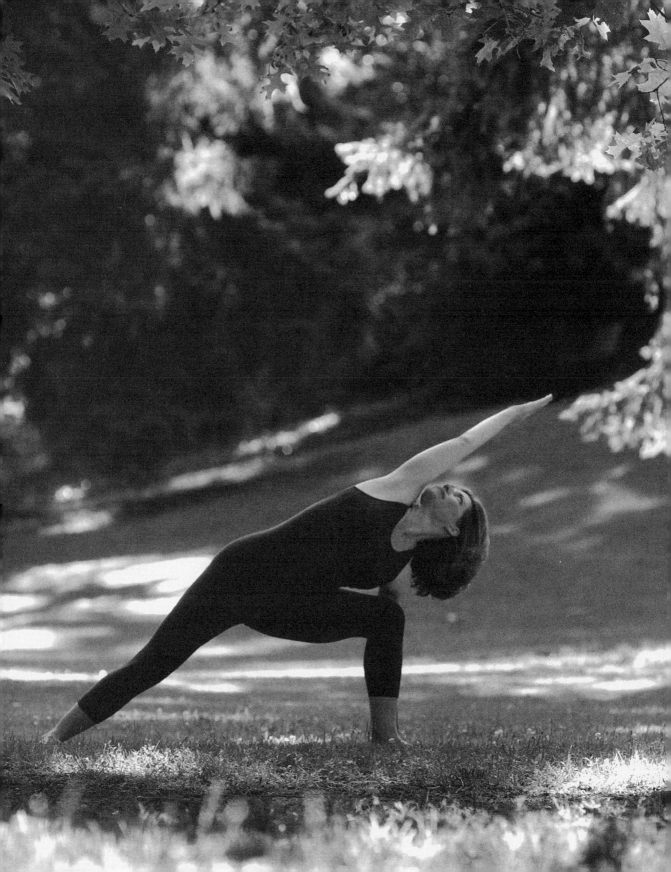

Lack of flexibility, not lack of strength, is what constrains most of us in Parsvakonasana. Placing the hand on the floor can compromise the full extension—and the alignment—of the spine for those who do not currently have the required flexibility for the classic pose. This problem is easily solved with the help of a knee or a prop.

- Assume Parsvakonasana as described on page 104.

- From the hip crease, laterally lean over the bent leg but place your elbow on your thigh, just above the knee.

- As you gain flexibility, place your hand on a block. Adjust the height of the block as you progress.

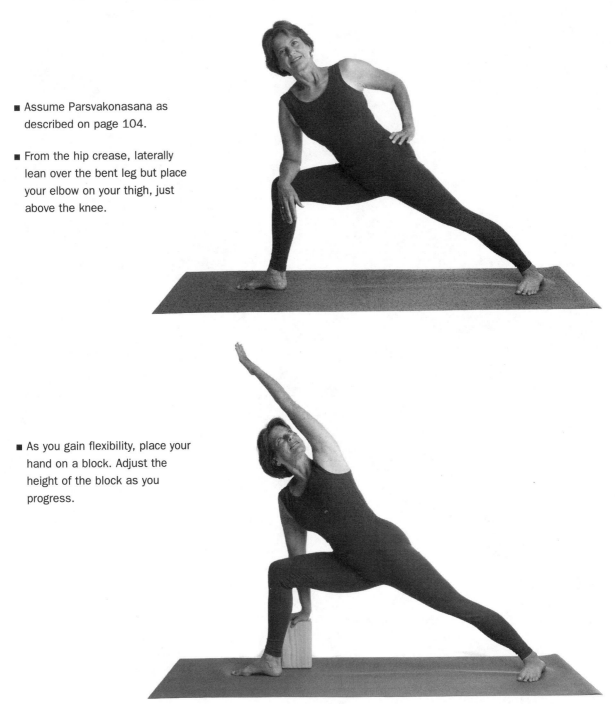

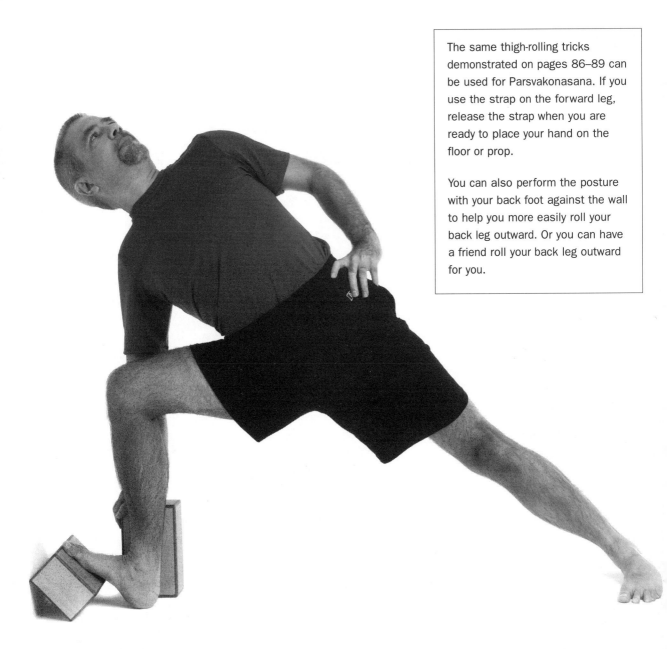

The same thigh-rolling tricks demonstrated on pages 86–89 can be used for Parsvakonasana. If you use the strap on the forward leg, release the strap when you are ready to place your hand on the floor or prop.

You can also perform the posture with your back foot against the wall to help you more easily roll your back leg outward. Or you can have a friend roll your back leg outward for you.

■ Prepare for the pose as you normally do, but with your forward foot on a slanted block, which is placed at a wall.

■ Place another block near your forward shin at the desired height.

■ Move into the pose slowly and carefully, as described on page 104, placing your forward hand on the block and your back hand on your hip.

■ Press your bent thigh and bottom arm into each other.

■ Notice how much easier it is to move your forward hip inward and how much more awareness you have as you move into the posture.

VIRABHADRASANA I
Warrior I

Virabhadrasana I, the first Warrior pose, is more difficult than Warrior II because it involves a twist of the torso without a full turn of the back leg.

- Stand with your feet four feet apart, aligned with each other and facing forward. Adjust your stance for your height.

- Lift your arms to shoulder height; keep your elbows straight and your palms facing up.

- Bring your arms overhead, placing the palms together. Or have the hands and arms shoulder-distance apart with the palms facing each other.

- Turn your right leg out ninety degrees and turn your left foot to the right by forty-five to sixty degrees. Turn your torso to the right.

- Make sure that you are aware of the four corners of your feet. (See page 13.)

- Lift your quadriceps, rotating your right thigh outward and your left thigh inward.

- Align your front hipbones by bringing the left hipbone forward and the right hipbone back.

- Move your tailbone downward, while lifting the muscles above your sacrum, and lift your abdominal muscles.

- Extend your spine upward.

- Expand your chest, lifting the sternum.

- Stretch your arms upward evenly from your armpits, but keep the tops of your shoulders relaxed. Soften your neck, throat, and face.

- Bend your forward knee into a right angle or as close to a right angle as you can.

- Maintain the outward rotation of your forward thigh and inward rotation of your back thigh.

- Gently bring your head back to gaze at the ceiling. If that action is uncomfortable, look straight ahead.

- Continue to lift your lower back and abdominal muscles.

- Stretch the back leg from the hip to the foot, pressing the back foot into the floor.

- Evenly stretch both sides of your torso upward.

- Hold the posture as long as you like. Release and repeat on the other side.

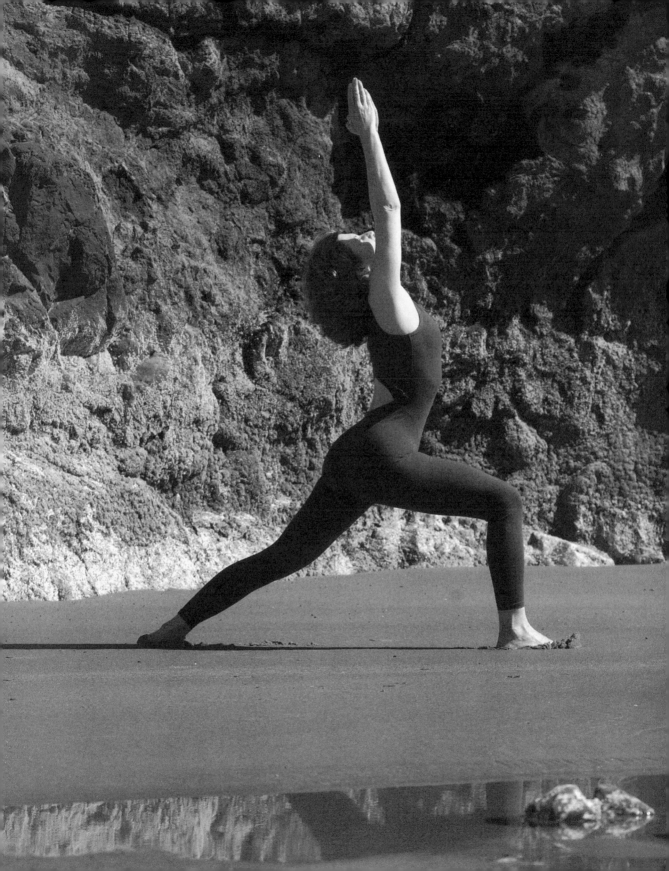

In the classic Virabhadrasana I, the torso turns without a full turn of the back foot and leg. Ideally, the hipbones should be even, which works for those with the required flexibility. For those without the required flexibility in the hips, a deep bend occurs in the lower back. This can tweak your back immediately or can cause damage over a period of time.

I have very stiff hips and have continually struggled with this pose. Once, however, during a yoga workshop, my entire pelvic girdle turned. Yes! The bones actually moved and I was able to perform the posture with perfect ease. For the next several days this miracle of the hips continued and I was so happy to be able to perform this posture correctly. Unfortunately, the blessing dissipated and I was soon back to my normal, limited hip movement.

In lieu of a miracle, practice Warrior I in this way.

- Stand with your back to a wall. Place the heel of your right foot against the wall and place your left foot forward three to four feet.

- Bring your right hipbone forward and your left hipbone slightly back so they are in the same plane.

- Place one hand on your lower back, just above the tailbone (or at the bottom of your sacrum), and one hand on your lower abdomen. Use the awareness of your hand on your back to allow the lower back muscles and tailbone to descend. The muscles above the sacrum lift upward. The lower abdomenal muscles lift upward and slightly in toward the spine.

- Lift your sternum and expand your chest.

- Keep your shoulders, neck, throat, and face relaxed.

- Press your heel firmly into the wall and continue to do so throughout the posture.

- Rotate the forward thigh outward and the back thigh inward—in other words, roll the thighs toward each other. (A trick for this is located on the next page.)

- Slowly bend the forward knee. It is best to practice with your leg in an obtuse angle while you build strength and flexibility. Do not bend the forward leg into a right angle if you cannot keep the hipbones even.

- Hold the posture as long as you like, release, and switch sides.

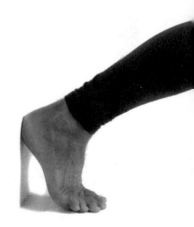

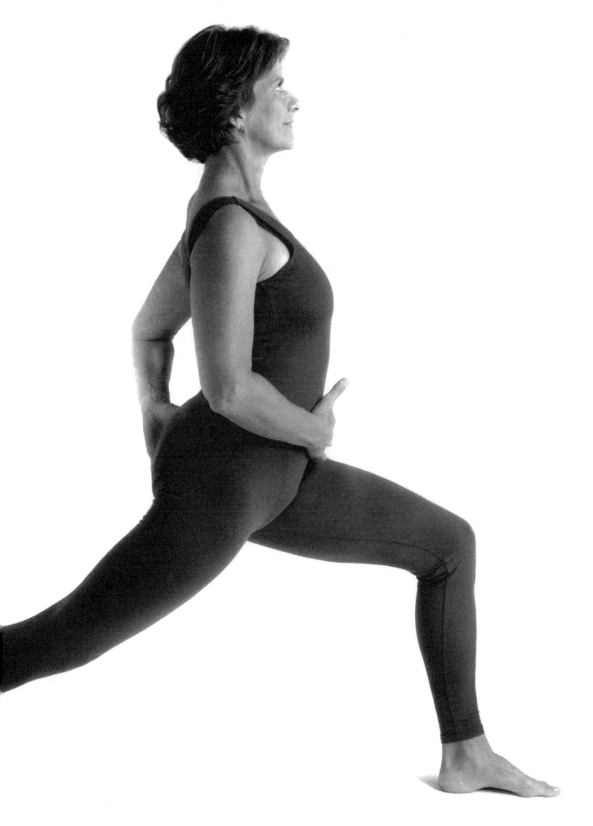

More than in any other pose, when I rotate my thighs properly in Warrior I, I feel tremendous energy moving up my spine. Rotating the thighs correctly allows the torso to lift more easily, building strength and creating freedom. Here's the trick that can make these things happen for you.

- Place a strap around your left leg, with the buckle on the outside of the thigh and the remaining strap falling outward.

- Place another strap around your right leg, with the buckle on the inside of your leg and the remaining strap falling inward.

- Place your right heel against a wall and your left foot forward by about three feet.

- Wrap the straps around your legs as much as you can.

- Pull both straps to the left as you bend your forward knee into Warrior I.

- Lift your lower back and lower abdomen and move them in toward each other.

- Keep your front hipbones even—or level—with each other.

- Hold the posture as long as you like and release.

- Switch the straps so that when your right leg is forward you will pull both straps to the right. It is worth taking the time to make the switch because this trick feels so great!

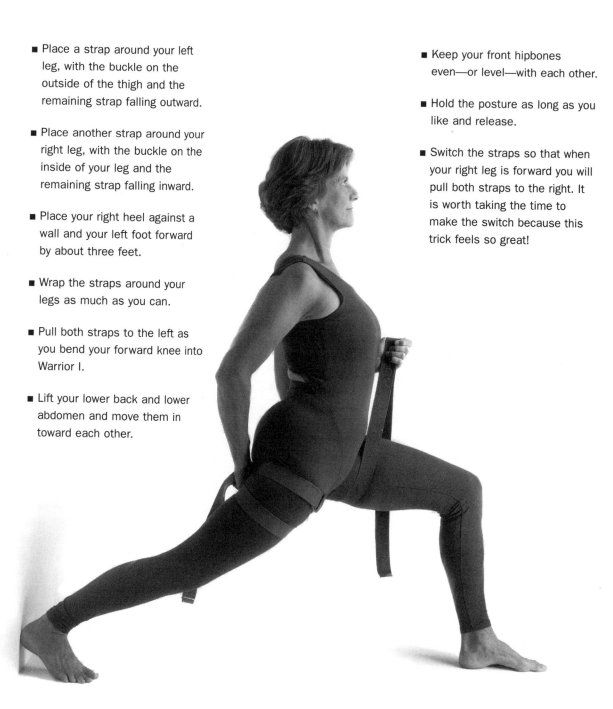

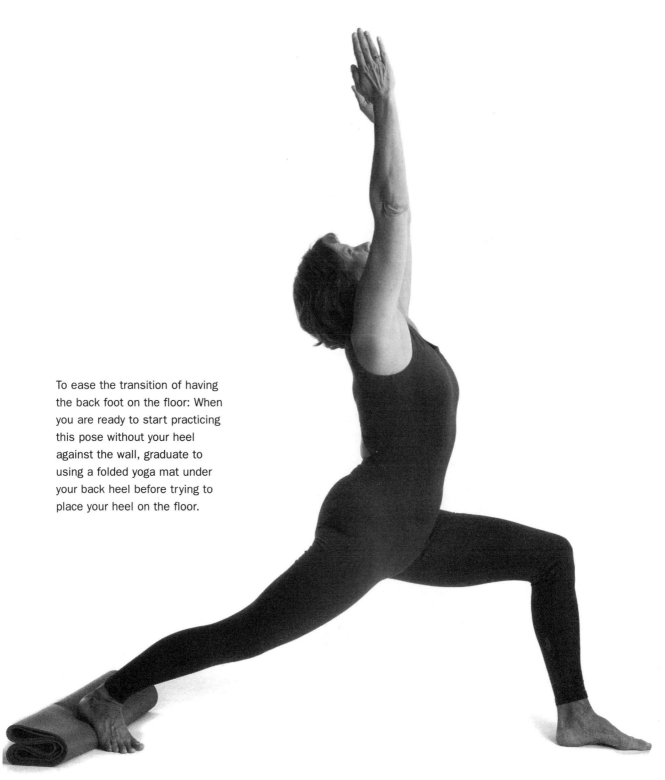

To ease the transition of having the back foot on the floor: When you are ready to start practicing this pose without your heel against the wall, graduate to using a folded yoga mat under your back heel before trying to place your heel on the floor.

Warrior I with Chairs

Lifting the lower back and abdomen is of utmost importance in Warrior I. As in Warrior II, if we rest in the lower back, we may ultimately cause injury and pain. If we practice mindfully we build strength, can correct our structural misalignments, and learn how to perform the classic posture in ways that are most beneficial for our specific needs. Here is a way to practice lifting your torso properly in Warrior I.

- Place a folding chair on each side of your mat.

- Assume the starting position for Warrior I. Lift your back heel and press it backward.

- Do a trial run, come into the pose and move the chairs so they will be directly on your sides while you are in the pose.

- Start over. Come into the pose and place the palm of your hands on the chair seats. Taller people can place their hands on the top of the chair backs but be sure to keep your shoulders relaxed. The tendency is to lift the shoulders when using the higher prop.

- Straighten your back leg, lift the heel, and stretch both the leg and heel backward.

- Press your hands onto the prop to help you lift and lengthen your spine and abdomen.

- Hold the pose as long as you like. Switch sides.

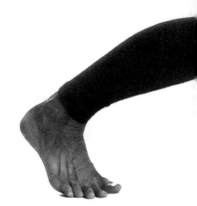

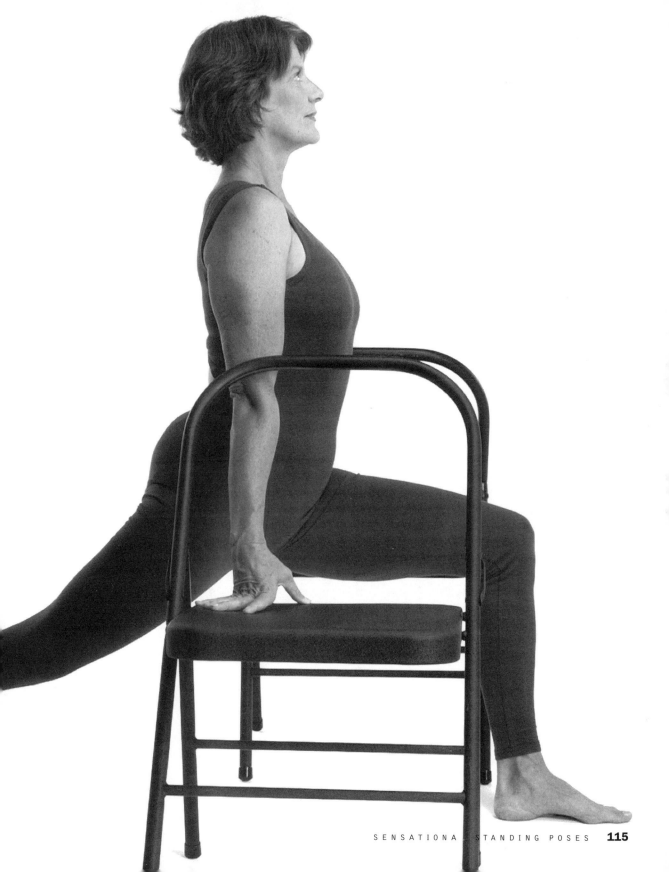

VIRABHADRASANA III
Warrior III

Virabhadrasana III is the most intense of the three Warrior poses, requiring strength, flexibility, and balance.

- Stand with your feet four feet apart, aligned with each other and facing forward.

- Lift your arms to shoulder height, with your elbows straight and your palms facing up.

- Bring your arms overhead. Your palms can either be together or shoulder-distance apart and facing each other.

- Stretch your arms upward evenly from your armpits, but keep the tops of your shoulders relaxed. Soften your neck, throat, and face.

- Turn your left leg out ninety degrees and turn your torso to the left.

- Turn your right foot to the left by forty-five to sixty degrees. Make sure that you are aware of the four corners of your feet. (See page 13.)

- Lift your quadriceps. Roll your forward thigh outward and your back thigh inward—toward each other.

- Align your front hipbones by bringing the left hipbone forward and the right hipbone back.

- Move your tailbone downward, but lift the muscles above your sacrum. Lift your abdominal muscles and slightly bring them in toward your lower back.

- Extend your spine upward.

- Expand your chest, lifting your sternum.

- Bend your forward knee into a right angle—coming into Virabhadrasana I.

- Lean forward, bringing your torso over your right leg, resting there for a moment.

- Straighten your front leg. Bring your back leg up behind you, to hip height, and straighten it.

- Keep your front hipbones aligned.

- Stretch your arms and torso forward. Stretch your back leg and foot backward.

- Lift both sets of quadriceps and rotate the standing-leg thigh outward and the lifted-leg thigh inward.

- Bring your lower abdomen toward your back. (Do not sink in your lower back.)

- Look forward past your hands.

- Hold the pose as long as you like, come back into Virabhadrasana I, then release the pose.

- Repeat on the other side.

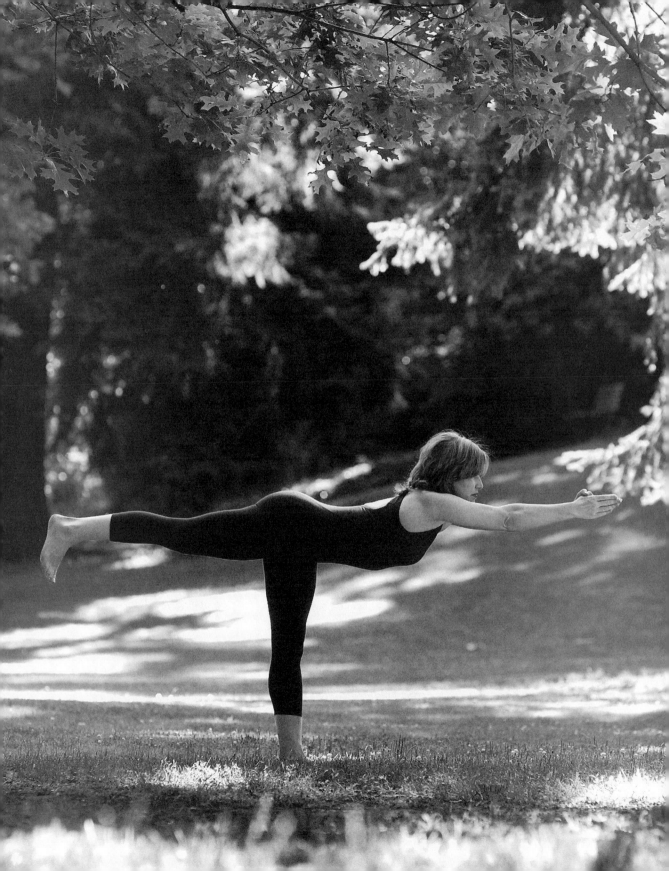

Performing Warrior III requires great strength, flexibility, and balance. Most of us do not naturally have those attributes; we have to work on developing them. The next few tricks will help.

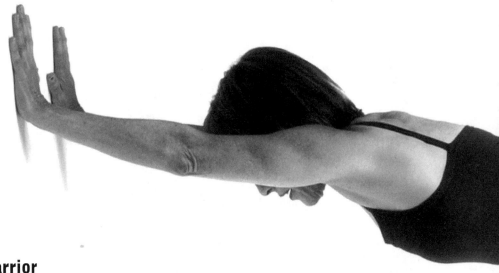

Right-Angle Warrior

- Stand very close to a wall and place your hands on it at waist height and shoulder-distance apart. (Make sure your hands are at waist height. Most of my students have no idea where their waist is!)

- Place your feet hip-distance apart.

- Walk back, bringing your torso parallel to the floor so your legs form a right angle with your torso. (See page 72.)

- Be sure that your hips, knees, and ankles are aligned.

- Press your hands firmly into the wall, straightening your elbows.

- Lengthen your spine.

- Lift your quadriceps toward your hips.

- Shift your weight to the right leg and bring your left leg up behind you so it is even with your hips. (The common error here is to have the back leg higher than the hip and that side of the torso slightly twisting up. It is better to have your leg lower than your hip than higher than your hip.)

- Keep your front hipbones even, in the same plane.

- Bring the front of your abdomen toward your back.

- Roll your standing thigh outward and your lifted thigh inward.

- Hold as long as you like and release.

- Reestablish your Right-Angle Pose, shift the weight to your left leg, and bring your right leg up behind you. Repeat all of the above instructions.

- When you are ready to completely release, walk in toward the wall prior to releasing your hands. Do not lift your hands from the wall and try to stand up while you are still in the Right Angle. That method of releasing could tweak your lower back.

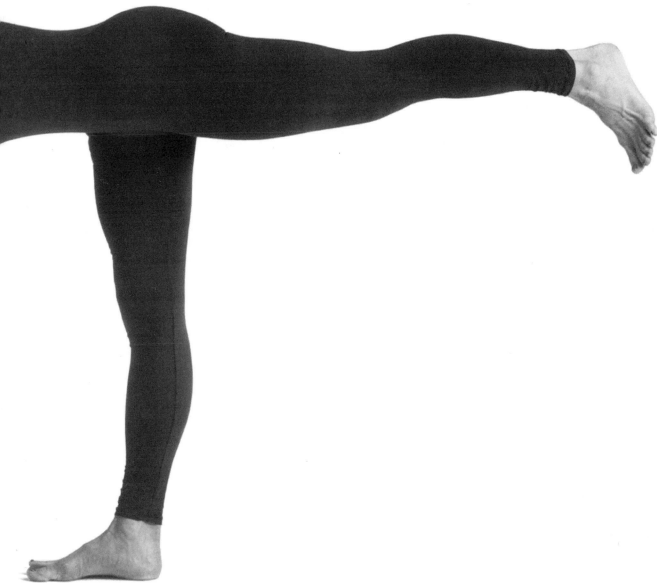

Supported Warrior III Tricks

In this trick, the wall helps you keep your legs firm and rotating correctly. It also helps you make the subtle movements that maintain the integrity of the torso. Having your hands on the blocks, with the torso and arms parallel to the floor, allows you to gain some strength and flexibility that are required for the classic posture.

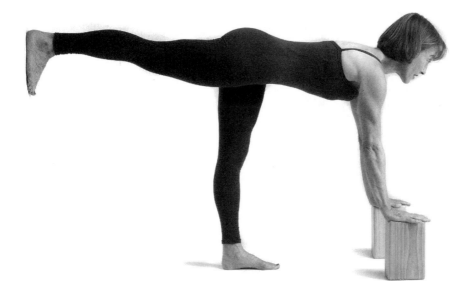

- Place two blocks at their highest height near the end of your mat. Make sure they are shoulder-distance apart.

- Experiment with this trick a couple of times to determine where you and your blocks should be relative to the wall.

- Stand near the blocks. Bend over and place your hands on the blocks.

- Walk your feet back so they are about eighteen inches from your blocks and hands.

- Lift your quadriceps toward your hips.

- Shift your weight to your left leg and bring your right leg up behind you. Place the sole of your foot on the wall and press it firmly into the wall.

- Be sure to keep your front hipbones aligned and both legs aligned with your hips.

- Work on bringing the front of the abdomen toward your back.

- Bring your leg down, reestablish your beginning posture, shift your weight to your right leg, and bring your left leg up behind you.

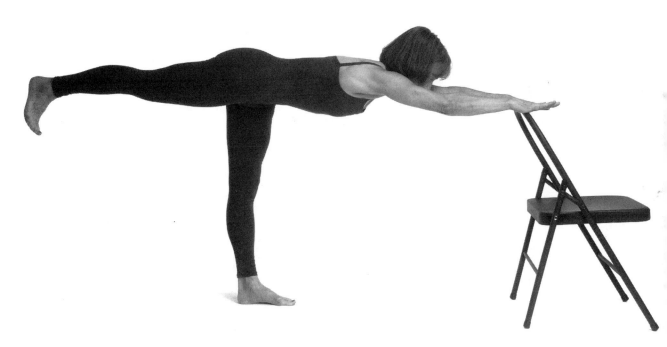

When you are ready to advance, come into Warrior III, as described on page 116, but place your palms on the back of a chair for balance.

ARDHA CHANDRASANA
Half-Moon Pose

Ardha Chandrasana looks graceful and elegant. Mastering this pose will help you embody these qualities.

- Start by standing with your feet four feet apart. Turn your left foot out ninety degrees and your right foot in ten to fifteen degrees.

- Moving from the hip crease, laterally come forward into Trikonasana and stay in this pose for two or three breaths.

- From Trikonasana, come into Parsvakonasana and hold for two or three breaths.

- Slightly unbend the forward knee and place the fingers of your left hand approximately one foot in front of you and a few inches to the side.

- Straighten your forward leg and at the same time lift your back leg so it is aligned with your hip.

- Lift your quadriceps throughout this action.

- Stretch the extended leg and foot away from your torso.

- Roll the standing thigh inward and the thigh of your extended leg outward.

- Press your forward hip deep into your body and keep it moving inward throughout the posture.

- Press the front of each thigh toward the back of the thigh. In other words, ground the femur bones deep into the backs of the thighs.

- Rotate the torso slightly backward.

- Extend the spine and torso uniformly.

- Bring your right arm overhead, align it with your shoulder, and slightly turn your head to gaze at your hand.

- Hold the pose as long as you like.

- To come out of the pose, bend the forward leg and lower the back leg and return to Parsvakonasana.

- From Parsvakonasana, straighten your forward leg and come into Trikonasana.

- Release Trikonasana.

- Repeat the pose on the other side.

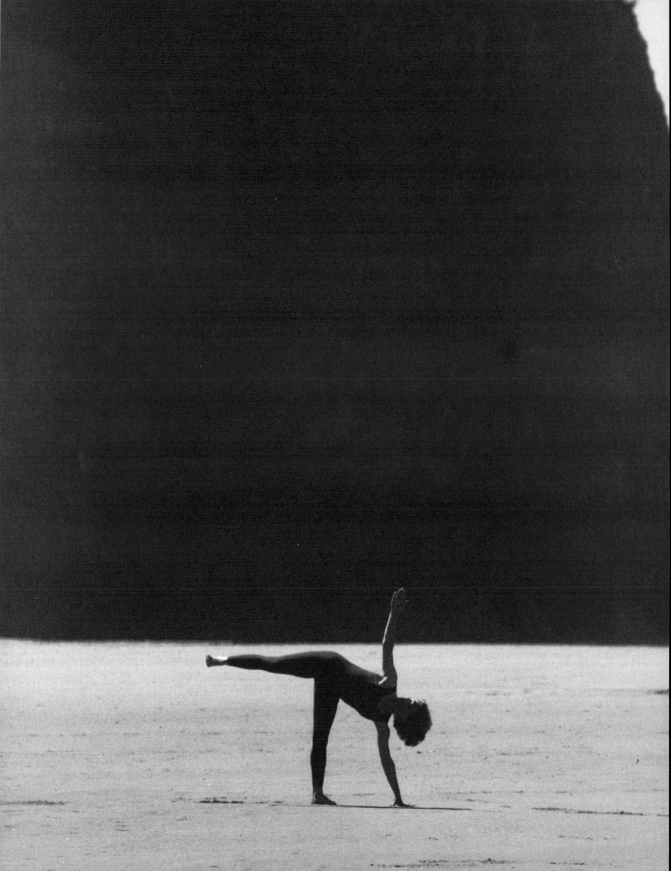

Ardha Chandrasana—Half-Moon Pose—requires an ability to flow into three poses. But many of us don't flow easily into Trikonasana or Parsvakonasana. Try these tricks to help you master Ardha Chandrasana, and in the process, master the other two poses as well.

Ardha Chandrasana at the Wall

Use a wall to help you balance while practicing this posture. That way, you are sure not to lose your balance. Use a block or a chair seat to help you get into the pose, if necessary. Make sure you have a lot of wall space.

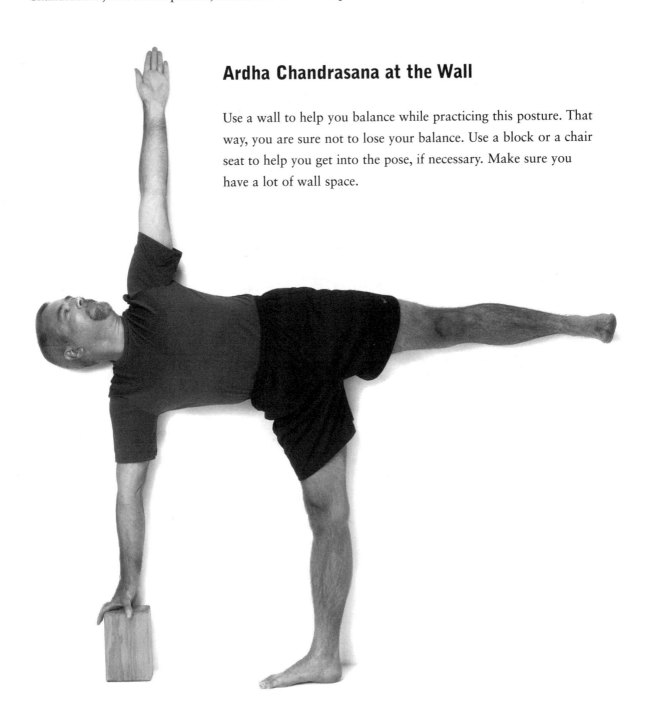

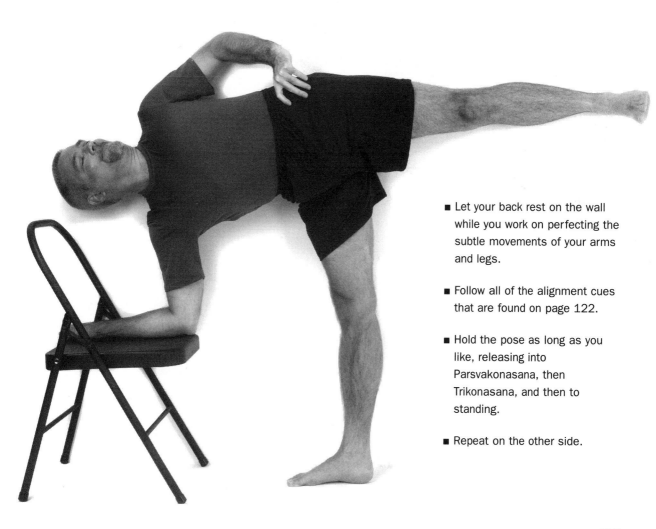

- Stand with your back against the wall. Use the prop that is most suitable for your current abilities. Remember that you will have to move the prop approximately a foot forward as you come into the final phase of the pose.

- Come into Trikonasana and then into Parsvakonasana.

- Let your back rest on the wall while you work on perfecting the subtle movements of your arms and legs.

- Follow all of the alignment cues that are found on page 122.

- Hold the pose as long as you like, releasing into Parsvakonasana, then Trikonasana, and then to standing.

- Repeat on the other side.

Ardha Chandrasana with Back Foot on Wall

In this trick, the wall steadies your back leg so you can more easily balance. Then you can practice the subtle movements of the pose. When coming into this posture, you cannot perform the pose classically because if you did, you would not end up with your foot on the wall. So try it this way.

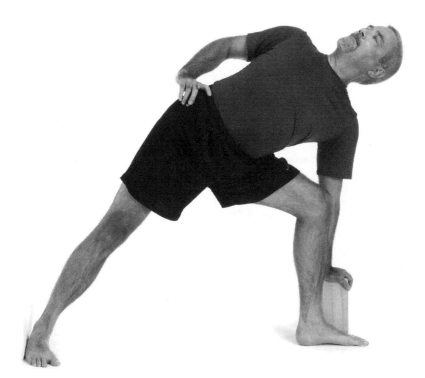

- Assume the starting position you would to perform Parsvakonasana, with your back foot against a wall and a block on the outside of your forward foot. Your stance should be a few inches shorter than your normal stance.

- Come into modified Parsvakonasana, placing your hand on the block.

- Stay in this pose for a few moments.

- Bring your block forward a few inches and slightly to the outside of your foot.

- Bring the back foot up the wall so it is aligned with your hip and simultaneously straighten both legs.

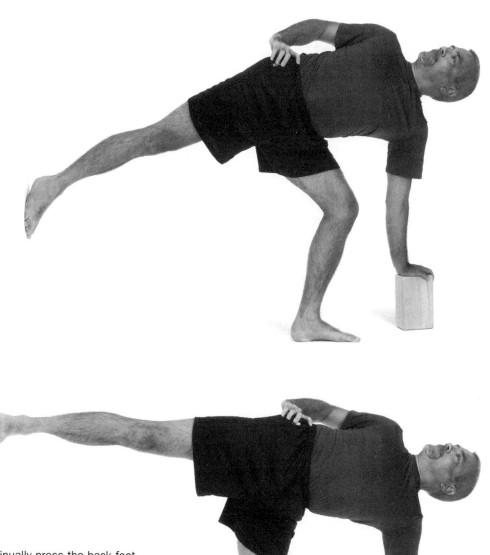

- Continually press the back foot into the wall.

- Follow the alignment instructions on page 122.

- Hold as long as you like. Release and switch sides.

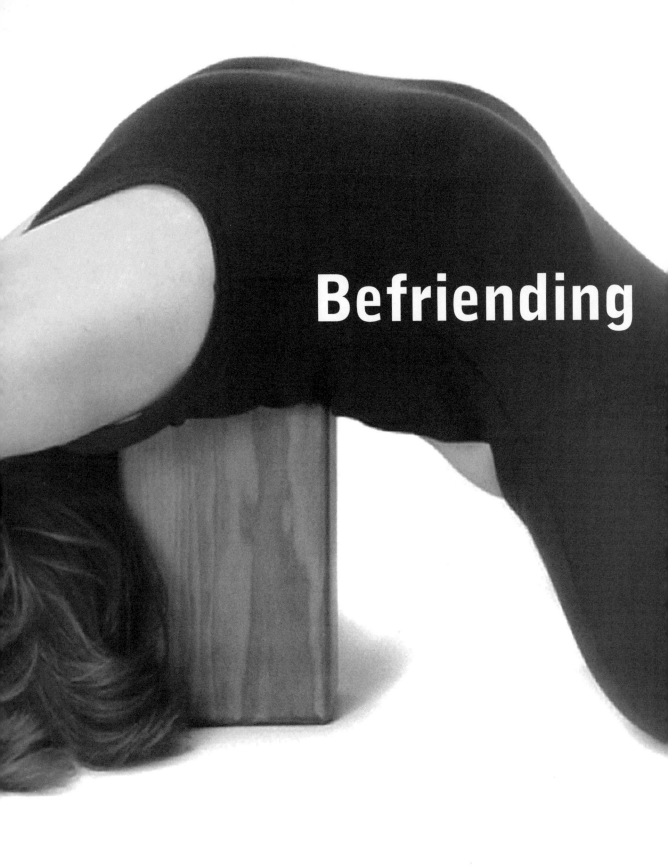

Befriending

Back Bends

Back bends tone the spine by stretching it. The back is strengthened and the whole body becomes strong, flexible, and supple. The chest is fully opened and expanded, which helps to cure respiratory illnesses. Back bends improve circulation and make us feel exhilarated.

The widespread photographs of gorgeous, rubber-limbed models in intense back bends may have given rise to the conception that you have to be a human pretzel to practice yoga. How often have you been amazed when you see these photos and wondered, Will I ever be able to do that? or, I could never do *that*! If you are identifying with this wonderment, this chapter is for you. In it is a broad spectrum of tricks that will allow you to practice back bends even if you don't have much flexibility, and some tricks to help you increase your pretzebility.

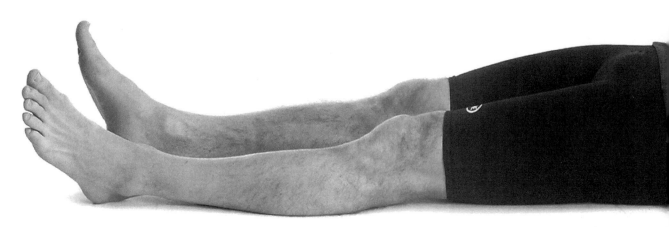

PREPARING FOR BACK BENDS

Back bends require tremendous strength and flexibility. Standing poses and inversions help you gain much of the required stamina and suppleness, particularly in your legs, hips, lower back, and upper body. For most students, their chests and backs are not able to arch as much as required in active back-bending postures. Forcing the chest to open only leads to injury. The body must, therefore, be prepared for active arching poses by performing passive back bends.

To open your chest gently and gradually, try any or all of these tricks. These are particularly good for those with respiratory problems and for people who are new to yoga. They are extremely relaxing and can also be performed when you are tired or when you have a headache, cold, or other illness.

Blanket Bends

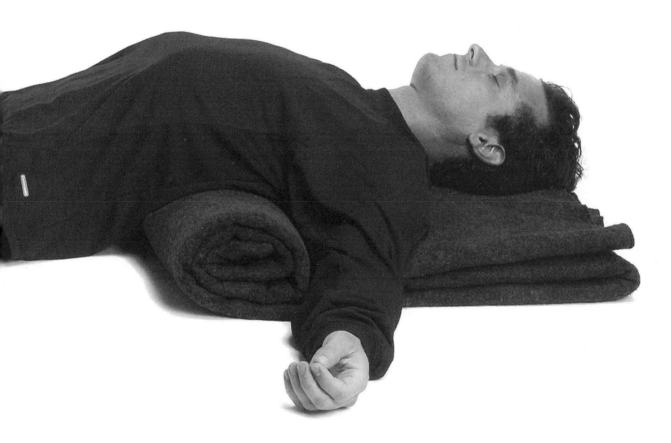

Roll a blanket and lie down so the
back of your chest is over the roll.
Your body is perpendicular to the
blanket. Support your head with
one or more blankets.

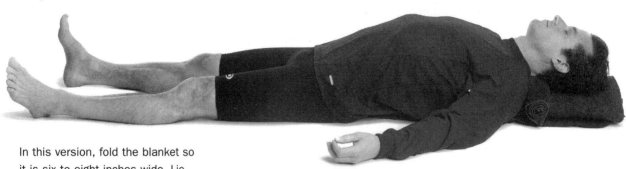

In this version, fold the blanket so it is six to eight inches wide. Lie down so the blanket supports your entire spine. Place a rolled hand towel behind your neck or support your head with a folded blanket.

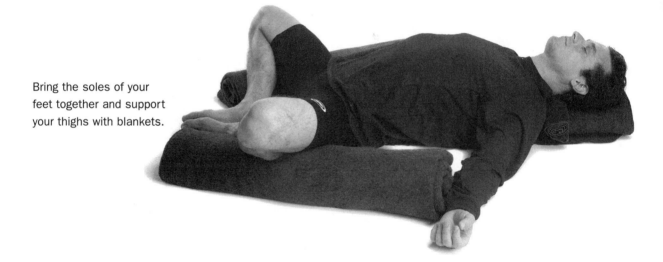

Bring the soles of your feet together and support your thighs with blankets.

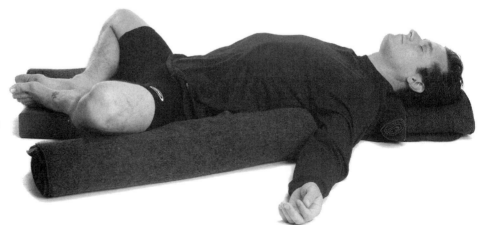

If your back is uncomfortable when the soles of your feet are together, place the sides of your feet on a block.

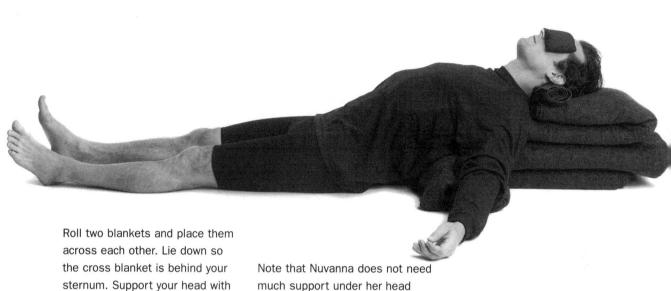

Roll two blankets and place them across each other. Lie down so the cross blanket is behind your sternum. Support your head with blankets, a neck roll, or a block.

Note that Nuvanna does not need much support under her head while Jimmy needs quite a bit.

If your back is uncomfortable with your legs straight, bend your knees.

Block Bending

Lying over a block can help open your chest and prepare you for traditional back bends. Start with the block at its mid-height. If that isn't comfortable, continue practicing the Blanket Bends.

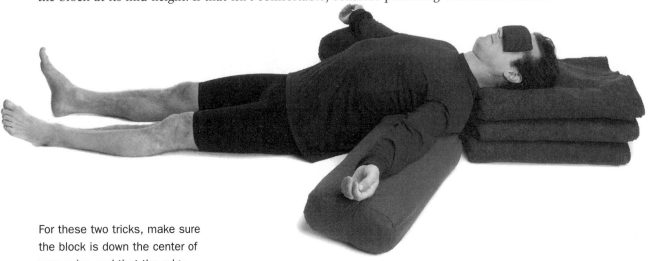

For these two tricks, make sure the block is down the center of your spine and that the edge of the block supports the base of your neck. Have your palms facing upward so the fronts of your shoulders can gently release. You can support your arms with bolsters or blankets, as Jimmy has, which is why you cannot see the block under his back.

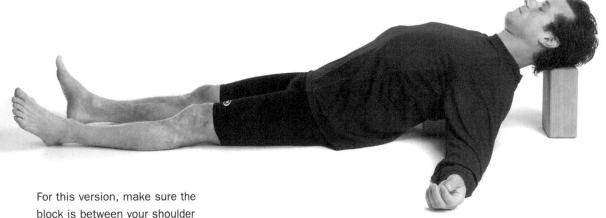

For this version, make sure the block is between your shoulder blades. Support your head with another block.

For these Block Bends, the block can be at either mid-height or its highest height. Make sure the block is directly behind your sternum.

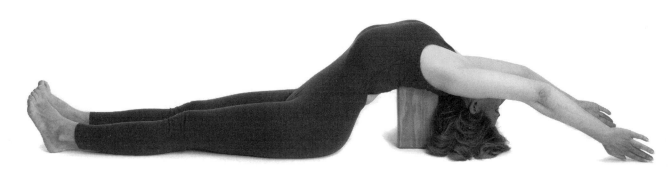

While lying over the block, you can extend your arms overhead and practice rolling your armpits and deltoid muscles toward each other. These movements are necessary in traditional back bends.

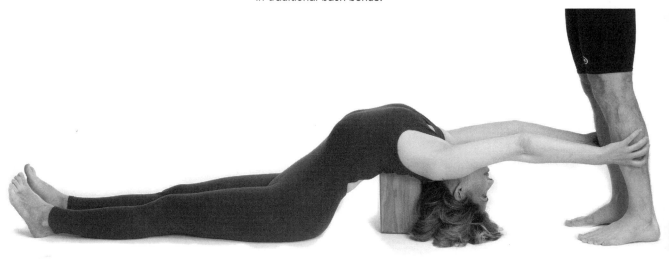

To help open your chest more fully and to practice rolling the outside edges of your armpits and your deltoid muscles toward each other, place your hands on a friend's shins. Have him walk backward slightly.

Back Bend/Forward Bend Combo

This posture is fun to try while goofing off with your kids or watching the nightly news with your honey.

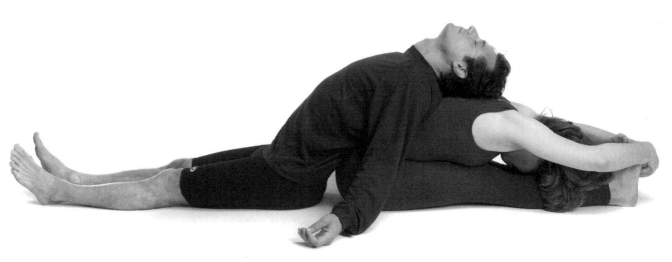

- Sit back-to-back with a friend.

- Partner A leans into a forward bend, while Partner B leans backward.

- Partner B, who is leaning backward, should completely rest on his friend's back.

- Partner A, who is leaning forward, may want to bend her knees to make sure that her hamstrings are not in danger.

- Switch roles, allowing each partner to try each version several times.

Airplane Back Bends

Every student I have ever had has loved this trick. I bet you will too.

- Partner A lies down on his abdomen and laces his fingers behind his neck.

- Partner B sits on Partner A's lower back, with the soles of her feet firmly planted on the floor.

- Partner B places the palms of her hands under A's armpits and lifts his torso.

- Hold until A asks to come down.

- Switch places.

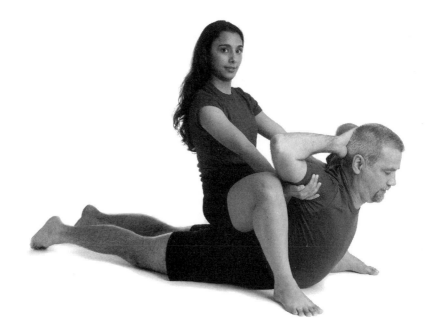

To further open your chest, try this Airplane trick.

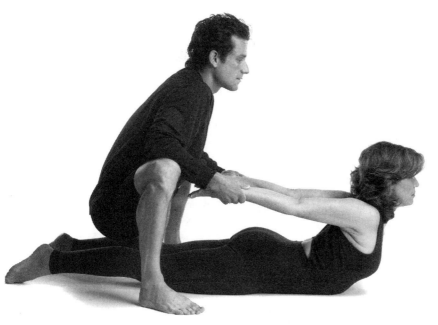

- Lie on your tummy and have a friend squat over your legs.

- Lift your chest and bring your arms behind you.

- Place the fronts of your forearms on your friend's palms.

- Press your forearms firmly into his palms, and have him press firmly into your arms.

- Make sure you are not tilting your head back too much, which could cause neck pain.

SETU BANDHA SARVANGASANA
Bridge Pose

Traditionally, Setu Bandha Sarvangasana is entered from a Shoulder Stand by dropping the feet to the floor and then making the appropriate adjustments. More commonly, however, the pose is practiced as a beginning back bend and is initiated by lying on the floor and pushing up. The second version is described here.

- Lie on a yoga mat with your knees bent and the soles of your feet as close to your hips as possible. Your knees and feet should be hip-distance apart.

- Lift your hips and clasp your hands. If you do not have the flexibility for this, keep your arms parallel and extend them toward your feet.

- Roll your shoulders under so that the tops of your shoulders are on the floor.

- Lift your hips as high as you can.

- Extend your hands toward your feet, keeping the elbows straight and the arms firm.

- Continually lift your hips and lower back toward the ceiling and extend your tailbone toward your knees.

- Press your upper and mid back toward your chest and expand your chest toward the ceiling.

- Firm your thighs. Press the backs of the thighs toward the fronts of your thighs and roll your thighs inward.

- Press the four corners of your feet into the floor. (See page 13.)

- Soften your throat and bring your chest toward your chin.

- Stay in the pose as long as you like. Release and rest for a few moments before trying again.

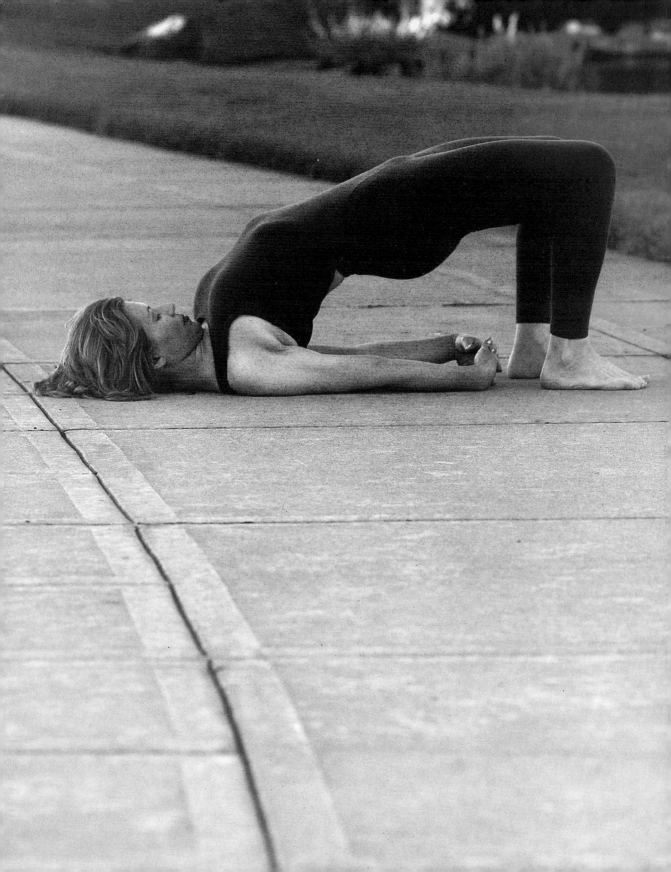

SETU BANDHA TRICKS

Setu Bandha is a back bend that can be performed passively and actively. In both types, we prepare ourselves for full back bends by opening the chest, working the legs properly, and increasing the strength and flexibility in our lower backs. Try some of these versions.

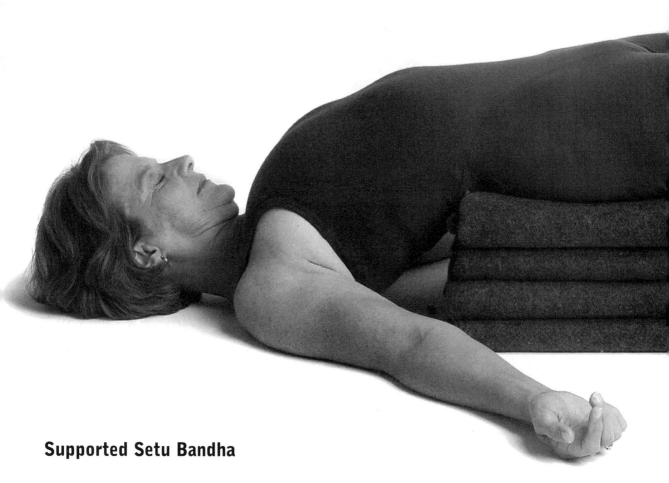

Supported Setu Bandha

These are the easiest ways to perform Setu Bandha, passively opening the front and back of the chest.

- Fold three to five blankets as shown. Fold them in quarters, and then in thirds.

- Place the blankets vertically on the floor.

- Sit on the blankets, lie down, and scoot your body off the blankets until your head and shoulders are on the floor.

- Keep your palms facing upward.

- Extend your legs and place your feet on a block if that is comfortable. If it is not, keep your knees bent and the soles of your feet on the floor.

- Stay in this position as long as you wish—using an eye cover and earplugs, to turn inward more completely.

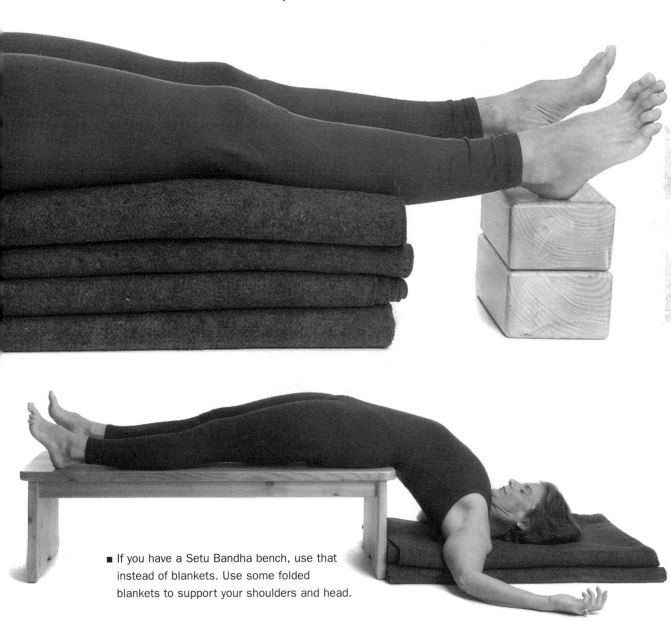

- If you have a Setu Bandha bench, use that instead of blankets. Use some folded blankets to support your shoulders and head.

Supported Setu Bandha with Blocks

Supported Setu Bandha can be performed with two different heights of the block. Start with the lower height first. If that is not challenging enough, place the block at its highest. Otherwise, start working with the lower height and, as you feel ready, move to the higher height. You can bend your knees or keep your legs straight. If you prefer straight legs, you can also practice pressing your feet against the wall, either at hip height or on the floor.

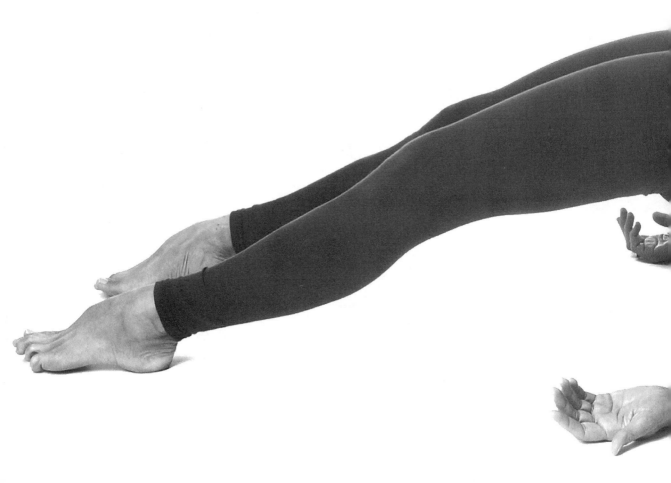

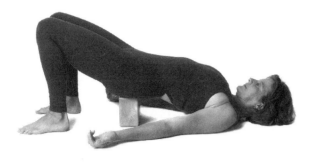

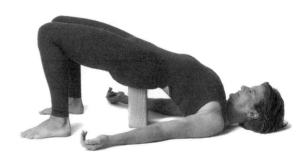

- Lie down on a sticky mat with your knees bent and the soles of your feet on the mat. Have a yoga block next to you.

- Lift your hips and place the block under your sacrum.

- Roll your shoulders under.

- Have your palms facing upward, clasp your hands, or place your hands on your back.

- Stay in this position as long as you like.

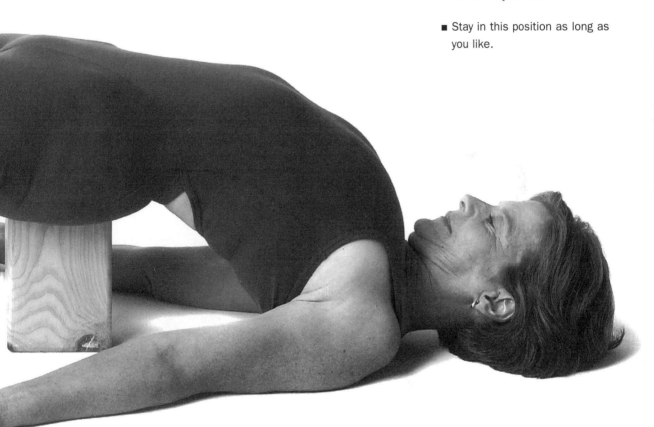

Active Setu Bandhas

With regular practice, Setu Bandha Pose builds strength in the lower back and legs very quickly. Many doctors recommend this posture to their patients who have back pain. To gain the most benefit, it is essential to lift your lower back to the absolute maximum. After trying these tricks, you will be amazed at how much you can lift. And your body's memory will help you lift higher the next time you try the pose without one of the tricks.

■ Come into Setu Bandha. Have a friend stand over you and place a strap under your sacrum and firmly lift your hips. Make sure that your friend's hands are low on the strap, close to your body.

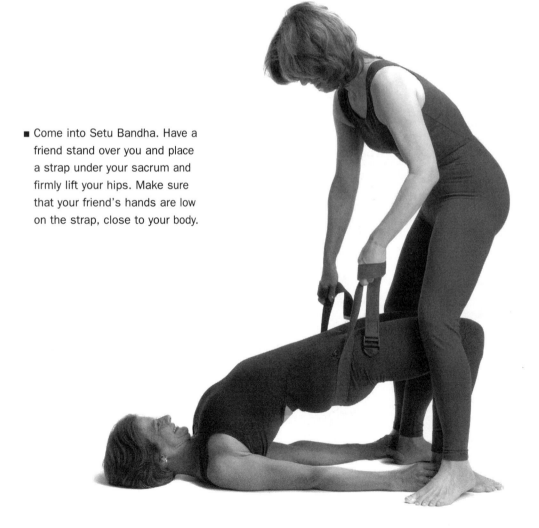

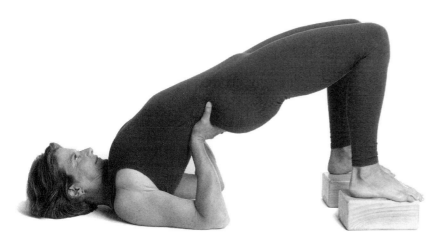

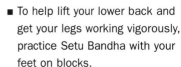

- To help lift your lower back and get your legs working vigorously, practice Setu Bandha with your feet on blocks.

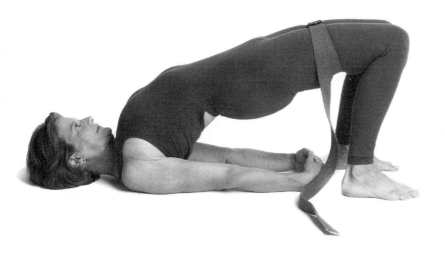

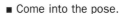

- Place a strap around your upper thighs, about two inches from the hip crease, and then lie down on the mat with your knees bent and your feet on the floor—both hip-distance apart.

- Come into the pose.

- Continually lift your hips and the backs of your thighs as high as you possibly can, as though you are going to break the strap.

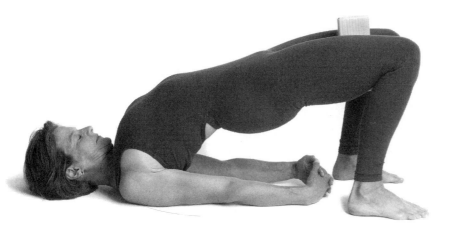

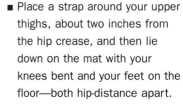

To really get the technique of rolling your thighs inward as well as lifting your lower back and hips maximally, place a block between your legs—at its medium width—and come into the pose.

Knee Pain Remedy

A common complaint from students as they perform Setu Bandha is that their knees hurt. If this is true for you, try placing a folded yoga mat under your heels. This trick has worked for all of my students who have tried it. I hope it works for you.

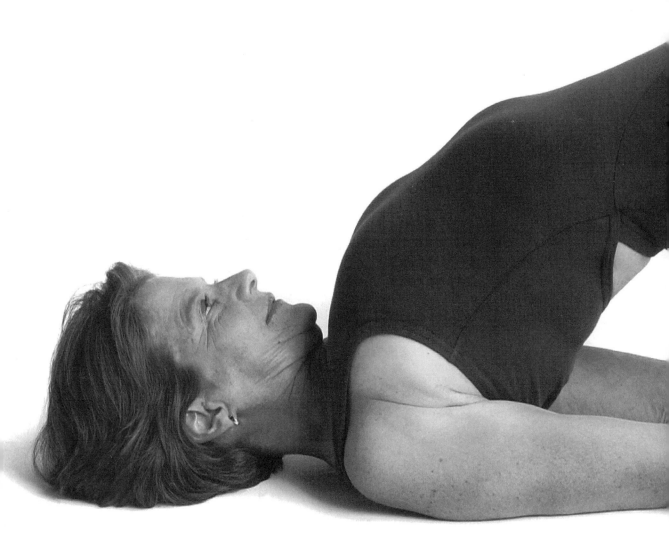

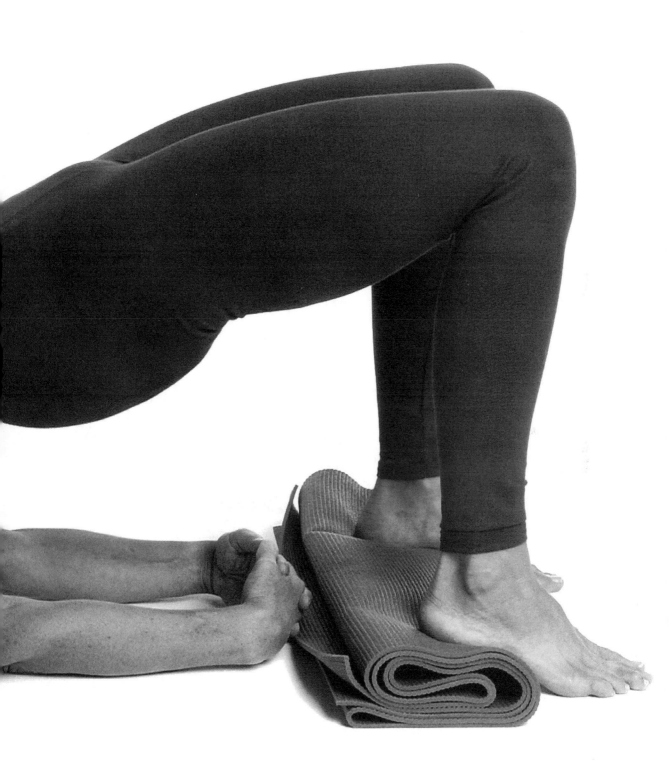

URDHVA DHANURASANA
Upward-Facing Bow Pose

Practicing Urdhva Dhanurasana, the classic Upward-Facing Bow Pose, is exhilarating and fun. It stretches the spine and helps us gain strength and suppleness. In this pose we fully open our hearts to others, to ourselves, and to the Divine.

- Lie on the floor or on a yoga mat.

- Bend your knees and bring your feet as close to your hips as possible. Your feet and knees should be hip-distance apart.

- Bring your hands overhead and place your palms, shoulder-distance apart, on either side of your head. Your fingers will face your shoulders.

- Lift your back off the floor and place the crown of your head on the floor.

- Keep your elbows aligned with your shoulders and your feet and knees aligned with your hips as you straighten your arms and legs. Arch your back and propel your torso toward the ceiling.

- Lift your heels and stretch your back and abdomen toward the ceiling. Then carefully place your heels on the floor, with awareness of the four corners of your feet pressing into the floor. (See page 130.)

- Throughout the pose you should:

  - Keep your weight evenly distributed on the arms and legs.

  - Press the backs of your thighs toward the fronts of your thighs and press the fronts of your thighs toward the ceiling.

  - Roll your thighs inward and stretch your inner thighs toward your knees.

  - Firm your hips and push your hips and lower back toward the ceiling.

- Curve the spine inward, pressing your upper back toward the chest and your chest toward the ceiling.

- Lift every arm muscle from the wrist to the shoulder.

- Roll the outside edges of your armpits and deltoid muscles toward each other.

- Slide your shoulder blades down toward your hips.

- Press the four corners of your feet firmly into the floor.

- Breathe smoothly and evenly.

- Hold as long as you like. Release, rest without doing any forward bends, and try again.

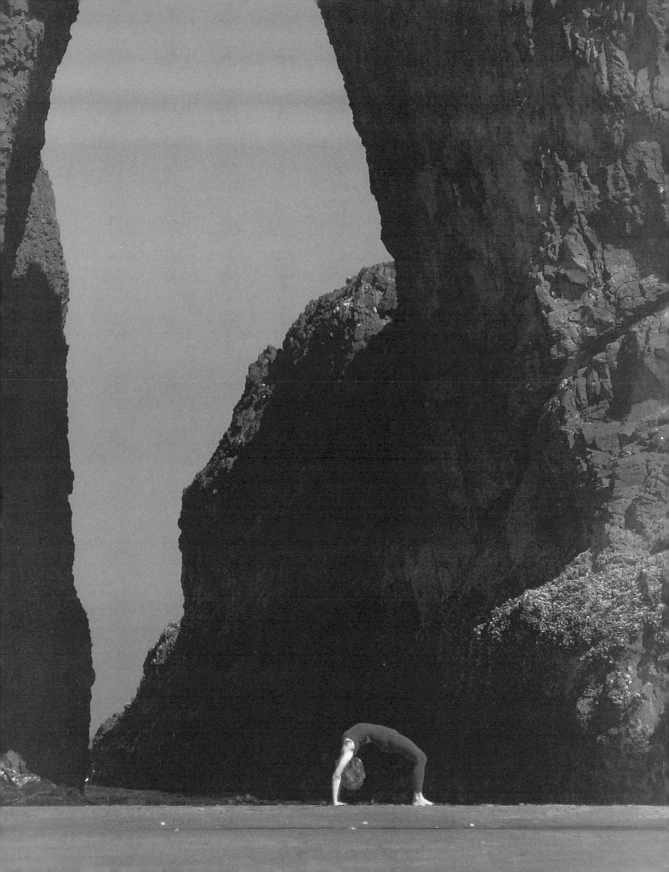

Urdhva Dhanurasana is one of the most exhilarating poses. I love it, but many of my students hate it because they simply do not have the strength to push themselves up into the pose. And those who have the strength often do not have the necessary flexibility in their chest, back, and shoulders. Thus, back bend–preparation poses must focus on increasing strength and flexibility in the arms, shoulders, legs, chest, and back. As always, practice standing poses, inversions, simpler back bends, and some of these tricks.

Chair Back Bends

The tricks, back bends over chairs, enhance your torso's flexibility. Some of them also help you learn how to make the subtle adjustments back bends require while your torso is supported.

Using the chair works for people of average and slightly less than average height. If you are tall, you can modify some of these poses by lying over a weight bench that has a yoga mat on top of it. With the weight bench, you can open your chest and back and work your arms and shoulders. However, the weight bench prohibits working the legs. With either the chair or the weight bench, try some of these cool tricks.

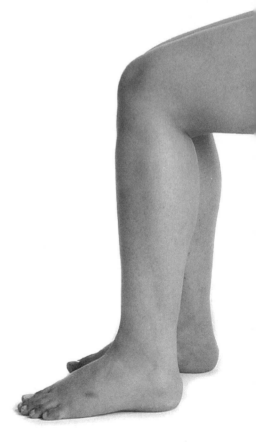

- Sit in a metal folding chair with your legs through the back of the chair.

- Scoot your hips through the chairback as much as you can.

- Lean back and scoot your hips through a little more. A good gauge is that the end of your tailbone is at the edge of the chair seat.

- Lie over the chair seat, making sure that the edge of the chair is at the back of your sternum.

- Keep your thighs at a right angle to your calves. Firm your thighs and roll your thighs inward.

- Breathe evenly and smoothly throughout each pose. If you forget to breathe, you may get dizzy.

- Firm your hips and extend your tailbone toward your knees.

- *Beginners should keep their hands on the chair.*

- As you become more adept, try the various positions shown. And for extra fun, try some combinations.

- To come out of the back bends, firm your legs and lead with your chest as you sit up. Bring your head up last. Rest for a moment by leaning forward over the back of the chair.

Hold your elbows and extend your arms overhead. Keep your legs and back firm but allow your torso to gradually relax and open.

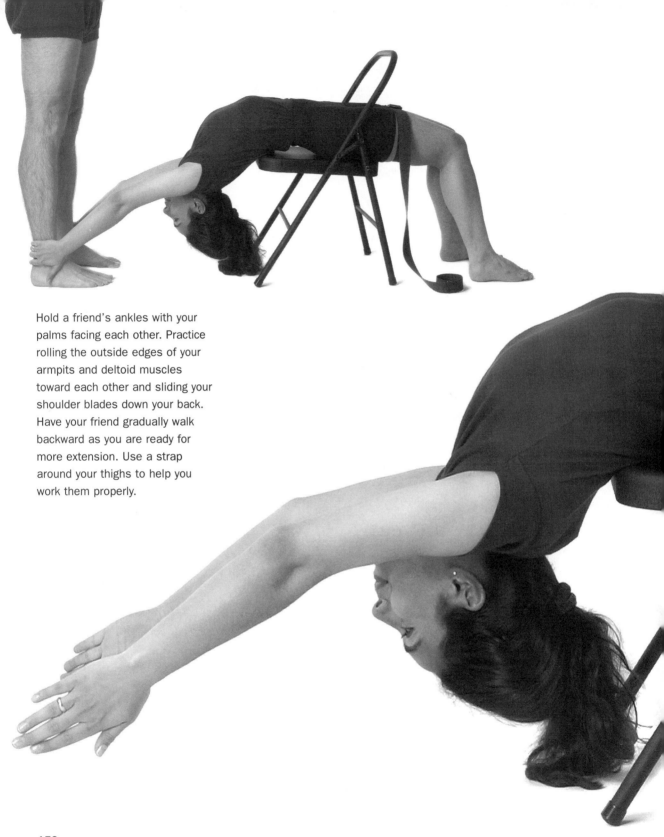

Hold a friend's ankles with your palms facing each other. Practice rolling the outside edges of your armpits and deltoid muscles toward each other and sliding your shoulder blades down your back. Have your friend gradually walk backward as you are ready for more extension. Use a strap around your thighs to help you work them properly.

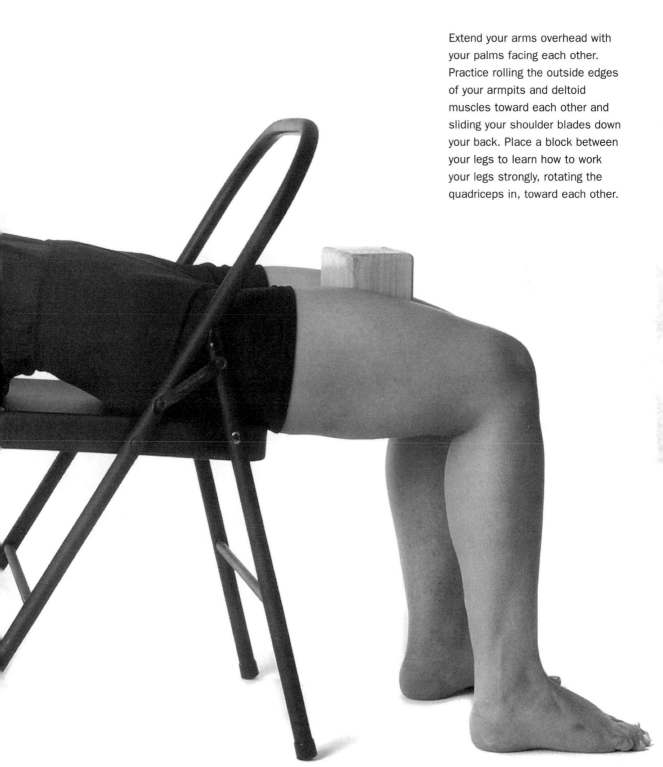

Extend your arms overhead with your palms facing each other. Practice rolling the outside edges of your armpits and deltoid muscles toward each other and sliding your shoulder blades down your back. Place a block between your legs to learn how to work your legs strongly, rotating the quadriceps in, toward each other.

Accessorizing Your Back Bend Chair

Accessories can enhance your chair back bends. The props encourage your chest to open more fully, develop more flexibility in your spine and back muscles, and prepare you for traditional back bends. As in the other chair back bends, scoot your legs and hips through the back of the chair as much as you can. As you lie back, adjust your prop according to the instructions below. The first time you try these back bends, hold the back of the chair with your hands and keep your knees bent. As you become comfortable with the poses, choose your favorite arm and leg positions. Stay in each pose as long as you like, making sure that you are breathing evenly. When you come out of the pose, sit up by leading with your chest and bring your head up last. Rest for a few moments by leaning forward over the back of the chair.

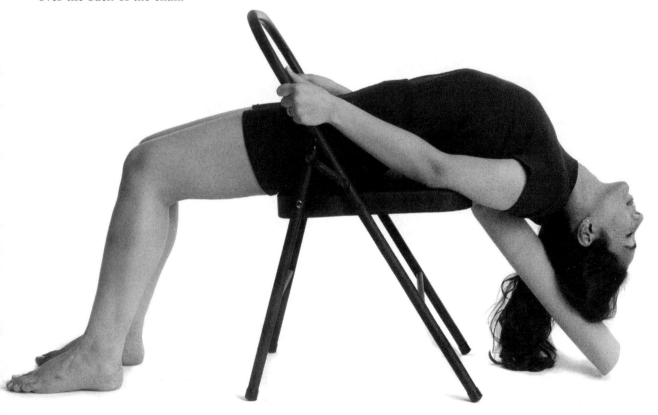

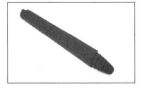

Roll a yoga mat as shown, with a tail at the end. Sit with your legs and hips through the back of the chair. Place the tail of the mat next to the end of your spine, *without sitting on it*. Lie backward, making sure that the mat is aligned with your spine and supports your head.

Fold a blanket so it is about eight inches wide and place it lengthwise over the chair seat. When you lie back into the back bend, make sure your spine is centered on the blanket. In this case, your head will not be supported so allow your head to hang and keep your neck muscles relaxed.

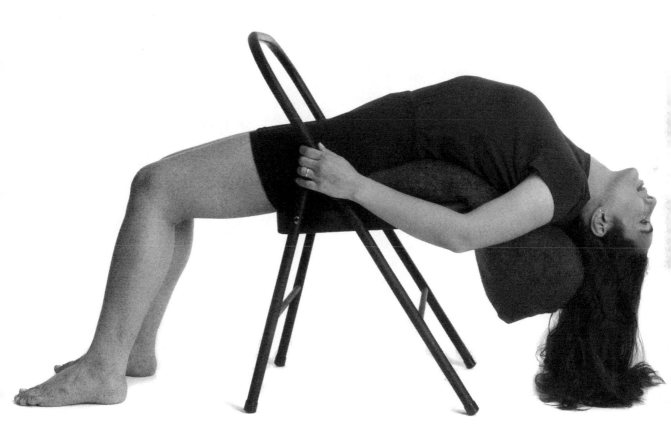

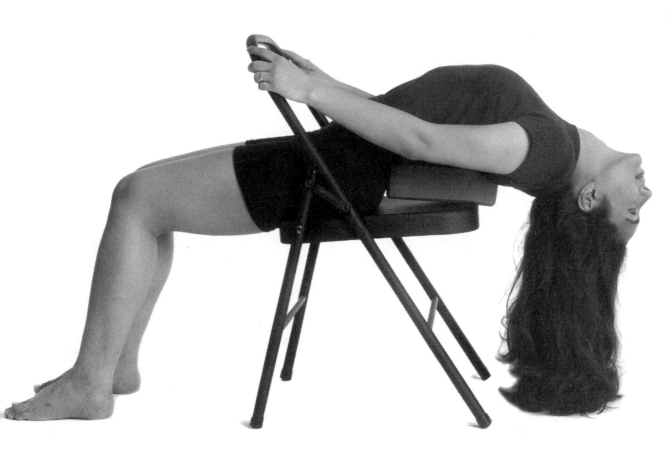

Sit backward in the chair and
place a block at its lowest height
behind you on the chair seat. Lie
backward and adjust the block so
it is behind your sternum.

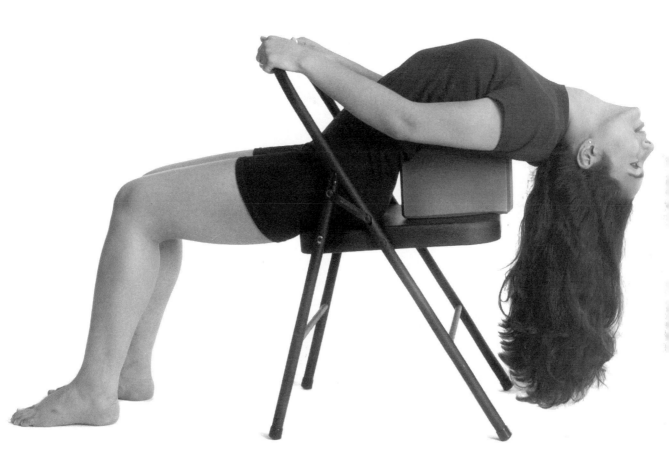

This time the block will be at its second highest height. Make sure the block is behind your sternum and between your shoulder blades.

Traditional Back Bends with Support

For those who have never attempted a traditional back bend, you *can* come up into a back bend with a little help from your friends.

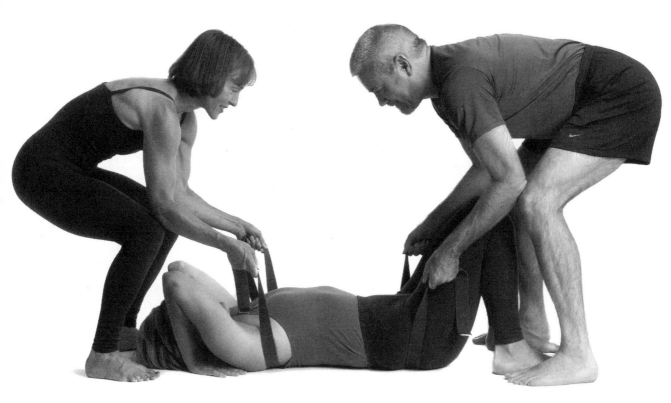

- This pose requires two helpers.

- Lie down with a strap under your lower back and another strap behind your sternum.

- Place the soles of your feet as close to your hips as possible, making sure that your feet and your knees are hip-distance apart.

- Assume the starting back bend position.

- Have your friends hold the straps close to your body.

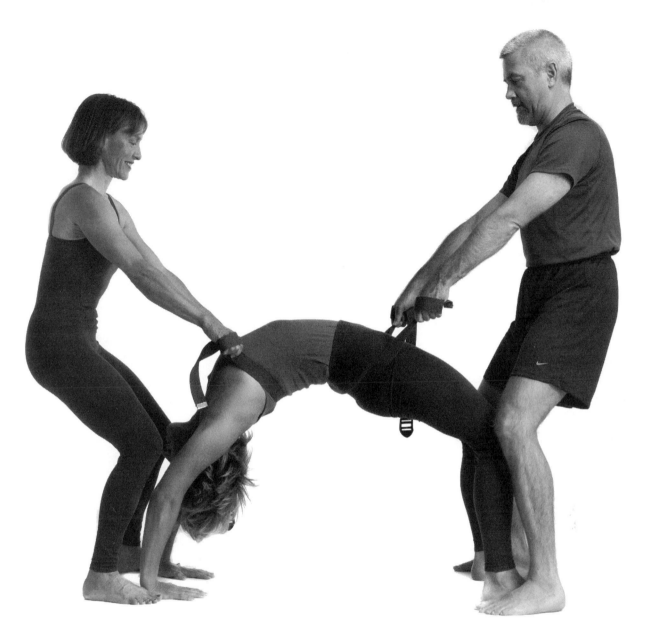

- Start to push yourself into a back bend as your friends pull you up with the strap.

- Be sure to breathe!

- Have your friends help you ease down when you are ready.

- Rest for a moment and try again.

Props can help us lift our chests and lower backs higher and more easily. They also encourage us to work our arms and legs properly.

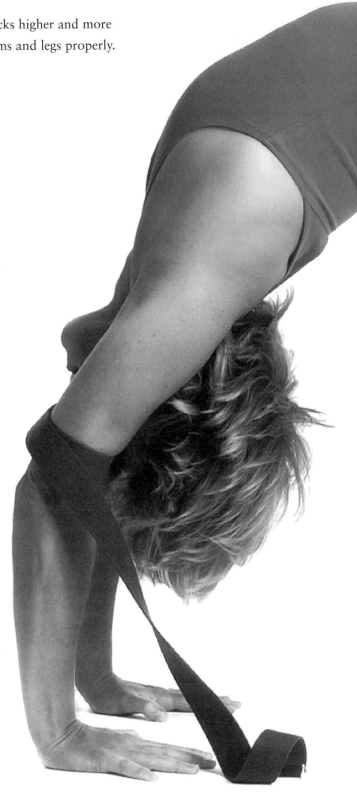

- To lift your lower back more in your back bends, place a strap around your upper thighs— about two inches from your hip crease. The strap should be taut enough so that when you pull your legs apart, your upper thighs will be about two inches apart.

- Lift up into the back bend and try to break the strap.

- You can also add a strap just above your elbows to help keep your arms in place. Tighten it so your hands and elbows will be shoulder-distance apart.

- You can practice with just the leg strap, with just the arm strap, or using both at once.

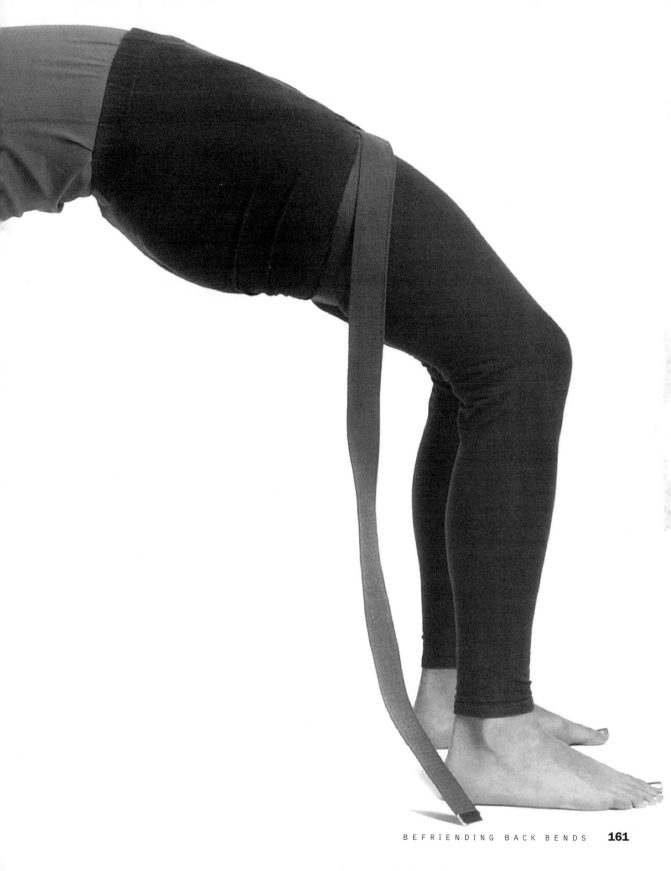

This trick gives you more lift in your shoulders and chest.

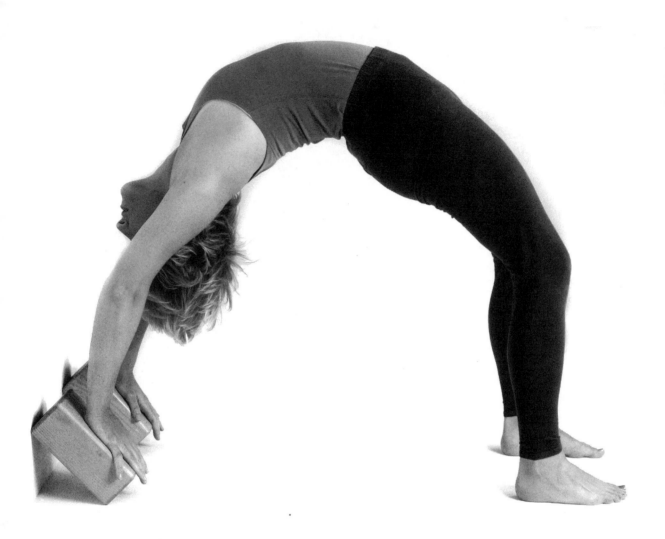

- Tilt some blocks against a wall.

- Come into Urdhva Dhanurasana
  with your hands on the blocks.

If your wrists are uncomfortable in Urdhva Dhanurasana, try this trick.

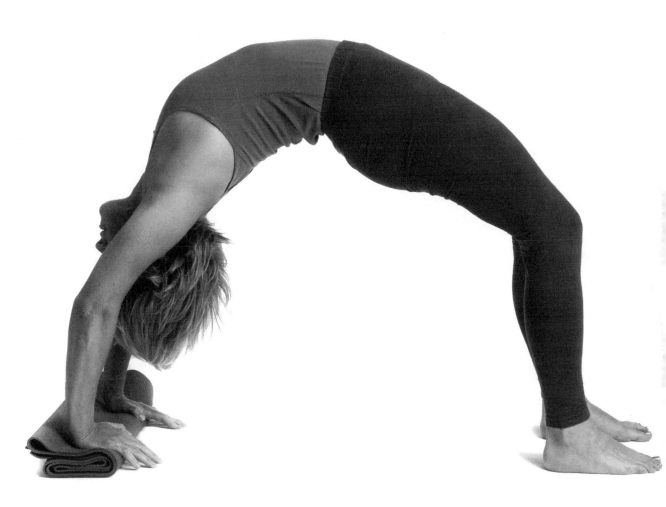

Fold a mat and place it under the
heel of your hands prior to coming
up into Urdhva Dhanurasana.

Arm- and Leg-Rolling Tricks

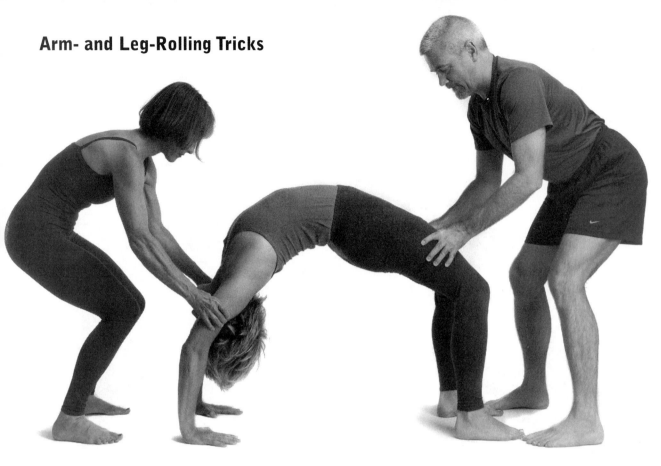

To help you roll your arms and legs properly, have some friends help you. Your arm-rolling friend should roll your deltoids toward her and your leg-rolling friend should roll your thighs toward each other.

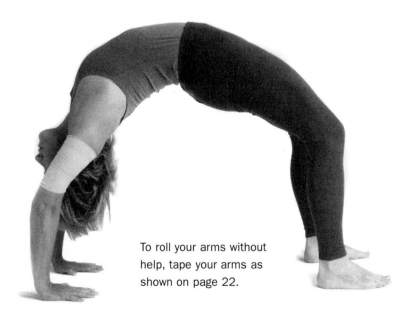

To roll your arms without help, tape your arms as shown on page 22.

Maintaining the Integrity of the Legs

For those of us whose legs invariably drift to the side in Urdhva Dhanurasana, which is usually caused by tight hips, try these two tricks.

Place a block, at its medium width, between your legs prior to pushing up into a back bend. The block also helps roll your thighs inward and enhances your ability to lift your lower back.

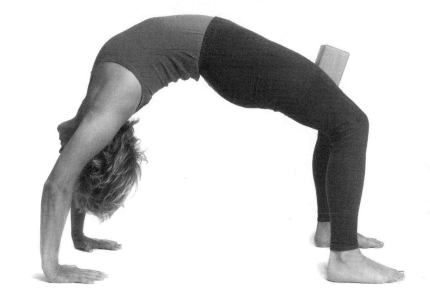

In preparing for the back bend, place a block, at its widest width, between your feet and press the sides of your feet into the block throughout the pose. You will be amazed at how well those disobedient legs obey the command of the block!

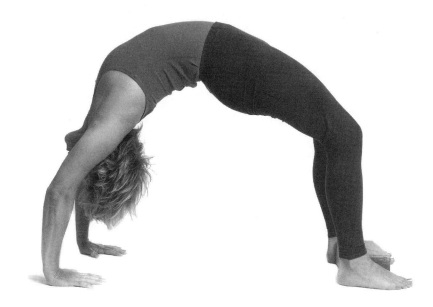

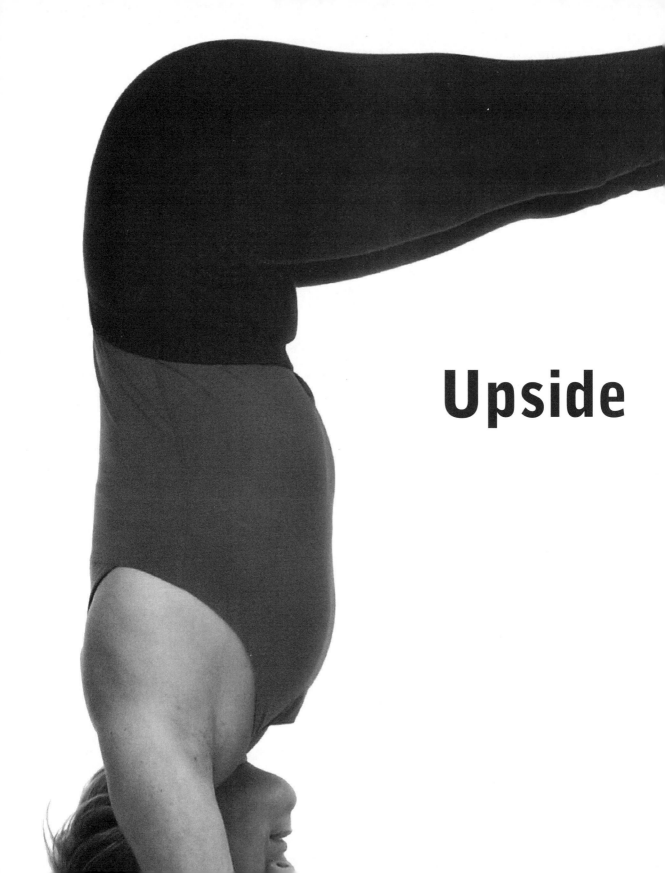

Upside

Inverted poses give us great energy. They help to balance the glandular system and the hormonal system, and bring oxygen to the brain. They increase our physical strength and balance. Emotionally, inversions help us find our internal balance and poise when our lives are upside down.

Down

Inversions give us new perspectives. When we see the world upside down, we glean new understandings. In a Shoulder Stand and Plow, our view is a more intimate one in that we gaze deeply into our own hearts. When you take the time to look and listen, what secrets does your heart want to share with you?

In inversions, we put our hearts above our heads. Can you imagine how our lives—how the world—would change if we all put our hearts above our heads more often?

ADHO MUKHA VRKSASANA
Downward-Facing Tree Pose, or Handstand

Handstands give us energetic joy, reminiscent of childhood. But with an adult body attached to that dynamic enthusiasm, take a few precautions.

- Place your hands, shoulder-distance apart, three to five inches from a wall. Make sure your fingers are spread and that your palms are firmly and evenly pressing into the floor.

- Walk back into Downward-Facing Dog. Establish a very strong Dog Pose.

- Walk your feet toward your hands. Lift every arm muscle, from the wrist to the shoulder. Keep your elbows straight and your shoulders lifted.

- Bend one knee and kick up, quickly following with the other leg.

- Place your heels against the wall and stretch the four corners of your feet toward the ceiling. (See page 13.)

- Engage your quadriceps, turn your thighs inward, and ground the femur bones inward.

- Lift your lower back and lower abdominal muscles and move them slightly in toward each other.

- Firm your hips and bring them into the body. Move your tailbone and sacrum up toward your feet and deep into your body.

- Roll the outside edges of your armpits forward, toward the opposite wall.

- Continually lift your arm muscles, shoulders, torso, legs, and feet toward the ceiling. Stretch both sides of your body evenly.

- Intermediate students can practice balancing by taking their heels off the wall.

- Stay in the pose as long as you like. For beginners, this may be only a few seconds. For intermediate and advanced students, hold for a minute or more.

- Intermediate and advanced students should come down slowly with straight legs, bending from the hip crease. Beginners, come out one leg at a time or the best way you can without collapsing your shoulders.

- Rest in Uttanasana for a few moments.

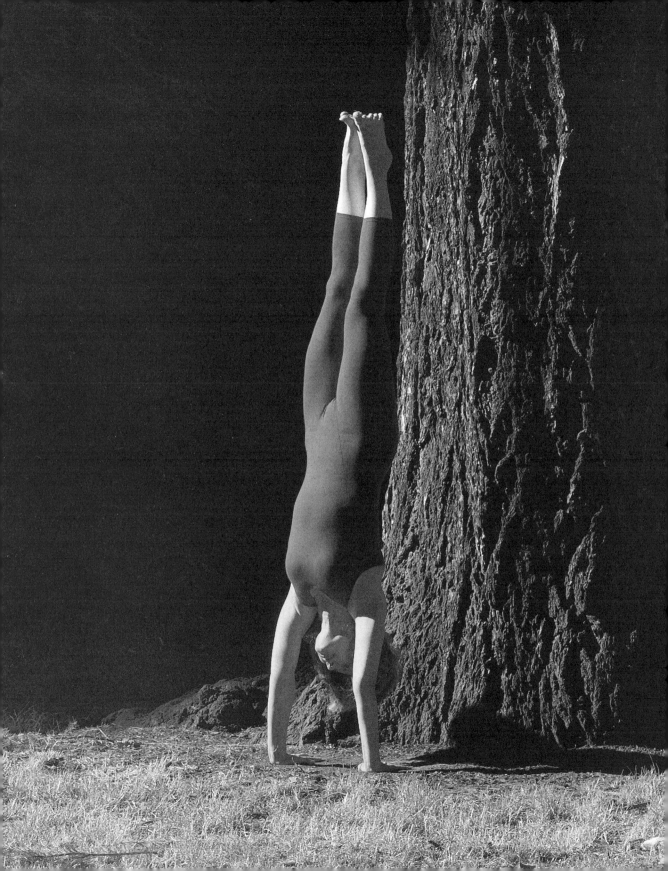

When women have trouble with Handstand, or most inversions for that matter, it is usually because of a lack of upper body strength. Lack of flexibility in the arms, shoulders, and upper back is what causes men to struggle with inversions. Other challenges students face in Handstand include lifting their wrist muscles, and poor stability and strength in their lower back and abdominal muscles. The following tricks will help you gain strength, flexibility, and proper form.

Right-Angle Handstand

This pose is good to practice to gain the strength and flexibility needed before attempting the classic posture. Have a friend spot you the first few times you try this.

- Sit with your back against a wall and your feet stretched forward.

- Mark where your ankles fall; turn around and place your hands where your ankles were, facing away from the wall. Make sure your fingers are spread

wide and your hands are firmly pressing into the floor.

- Walk your feet up the wall until your torso forms a right angle with your legs.

- Lift every arm muscle from the wrists to the shoulders.

- Engage your quadriceps and roll your thighs inward. Press the fronts of your thighs toward the backs of your thighs.

- Press your feet firmly into the wall.

- Lengthen your spine and stretch both sides of your torso evenly.

- Allow your head to hang, softening your neck muscles.

- To release, walk your feet down the wall. Lean forward in Uttanasana for a few moments.

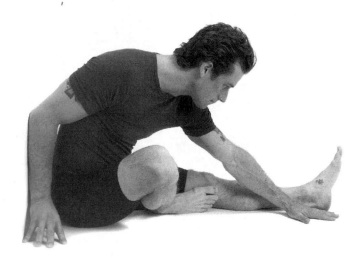

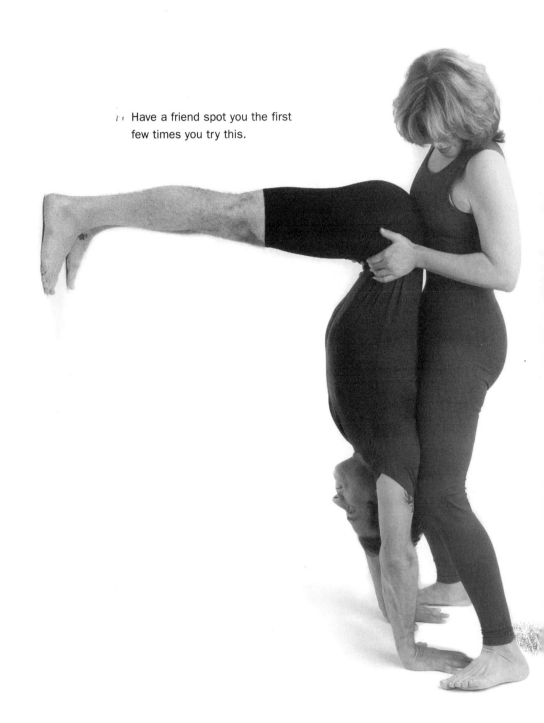

⌐ Have a friend spot you the first
few times you try this.

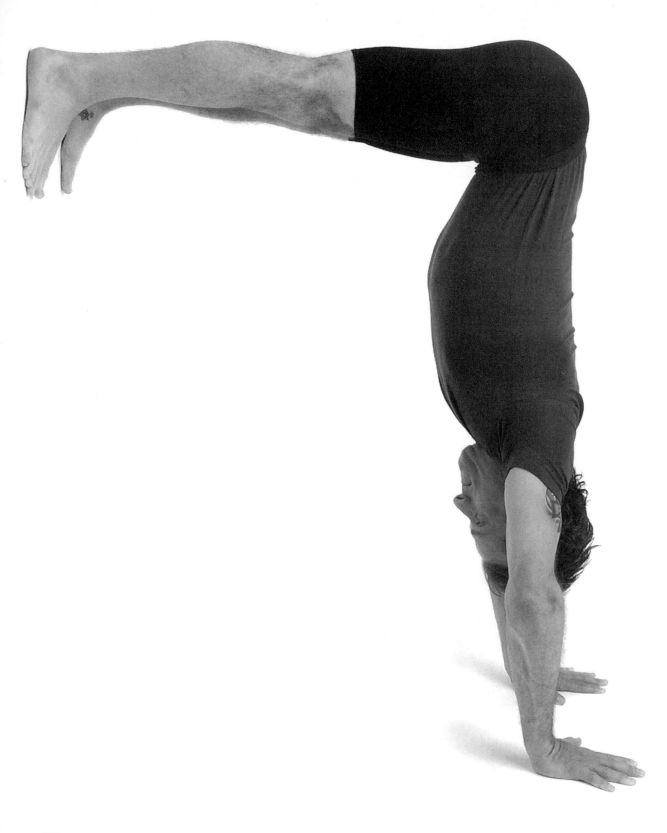

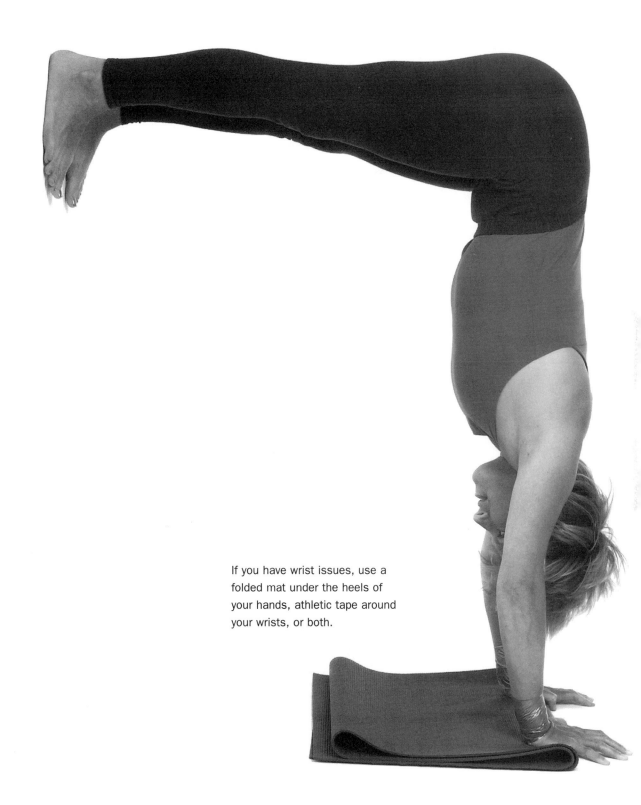

If you have wrist issues, use a
folded mat under the heels of
your hands, athletic tape around
your wrists, or both.

Full Handstand Tricks

Another challenge that many students face in Handstand is keeping their lower backs lifted. The danger of not lifting properly is that the lower back muscles collapse, or "rest," while upside down. This can immediately tweak your back or it can cause damage over time. To learn to lift your lower back properly, try the following trick. Pay attention to all of the aspects of Handstand, as described on page 168, but focus on your lower back.

- Come into Handstand as described on page 168, but bend your knees and place your toes on the wall. Firm your lower back and abdomen. Move your tailbone and sacrum deep into your body and toward the ceiling. These actions stabilize the pose.

- If you have wrist issues, wrap your wrists with athletic tape (as shown) or place a folded yoga mat under the heels of your hands.

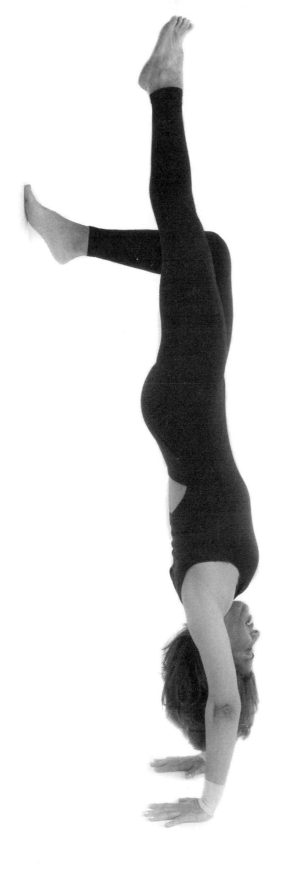

Practice balancing by bringing one leg straight up. Firm your legs and lower back. Practice lifting one leg at a time. As you are ready, bring the second leg straight up to join the first one.

PINCA MAYURASANA

Peacock Pose, or Forearm Balance

A regular practice of Pinca Mayurasana heightens our enthusiasm, exhilaration, and joy. Named after the elegant peacock, this pose enhances our sense of poise, balance, and grace. Note: Beginner and intermediate students should use a wall for this pose.

- Kneel in front of a wall and place your forearms and palms on the floor, facing the wall, shoulder-distance apart. You may want to place your hands around a block and use a strap around your upper arms to ensure that your arms and hands maintain proper alignment throughout the pose.

- Press your forearms into the floor. Pay specific attention to the insides of your wrists, which naturally want to resist that movement. So be particularly aware of grounding the wrists throughout the pose.

- Straighten your legs and, while lifting your shoulders to your absolute maximum, walk in toward the wall.

- Bend one leg, kick up, and quickly follow with the other leg.

- Place your heels together on the wall and stretch the four forners of your feet toward the ceiling. (See page 13.)

- Engage your quadriceps, roll your thighs inward, and ground your femur bones deep into your body.

- Lift your tailbone, sacrum, and lower back up toward the ceiling and move them in toward your abdomen.

- Tighten your hips and move them toward your abdomen.

- Lift your lower abdominal muscles and move them slightly in toward your back.

- Move your upper back slightly in toward your chest.

- Rotate the outside edges of your armpits and deltoid muscles forward.

- Lift your head and look forward.

- As you are ready, you can take your feet away from the wall and balance. Return your feet to the wall when you falter.

- Over time you will be able to enter the pose without the support of the wall.

- Stay in the pose as long as you like. Release and rest in Child's Pose for a few moments.

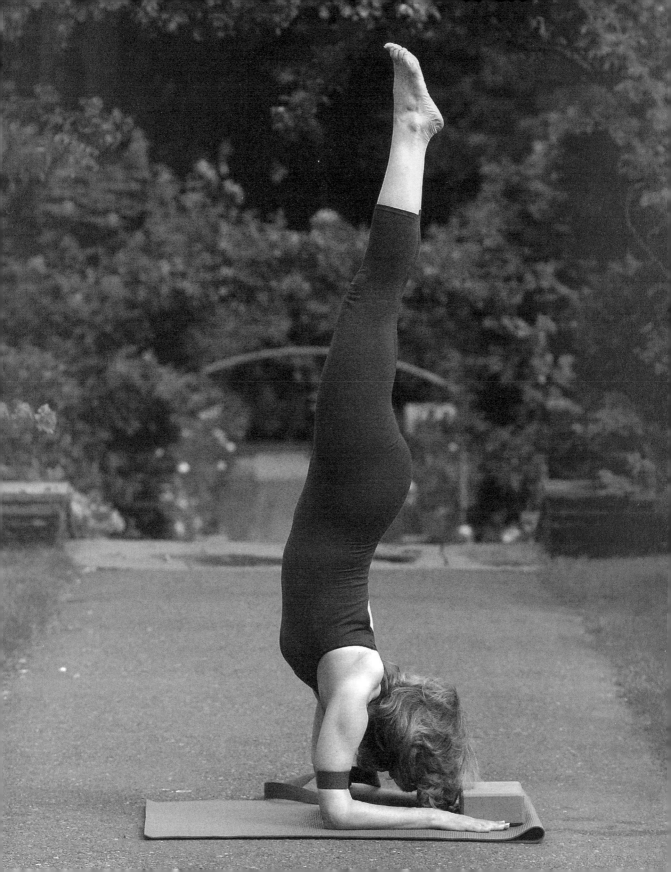

Pinca Mayurasana has many benefits and many challenges. Like all inversions, Forearm Balance energizes us, increases circulation to the brain, and enhances upper body strength and flexibility. The challenging aspects of the pose include:

■ keeping the hands and arms aligned with the shoulders

■ keeping the forearms firmly pressed into the floor

■ maintaining the lift of the lower back

In addition to these specific problems, this pose requires strength and flexibility in the shoulders and the upper body that most of us simply do not have when we start yoga. Bearing our own weight upside down is not easy. In Pinca Mayurasana, we bear that weight on our forearms while our shoulders are rotated in an unusual way. Therefore, it is absolutely necessary to lift the shoulders maximally to avoid injury. Following are some tricks to help with these challenges.

Come into the pose as described on page 176, but do not kick up. Place your hands around a yoga block with your thumbs in front of the block and your forefingers on the sides of the block. The webbing between the thumbs and forefingers is firmly placed on the edges of the block. I had to practice this version for many months before I gained the strength to kick up against the wall.

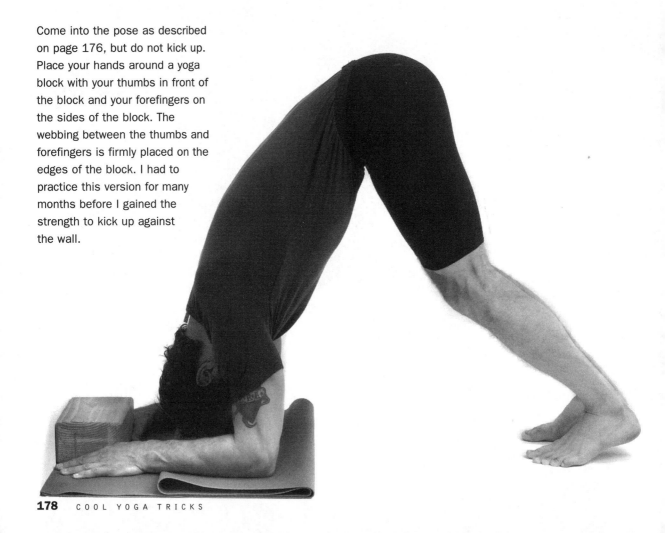

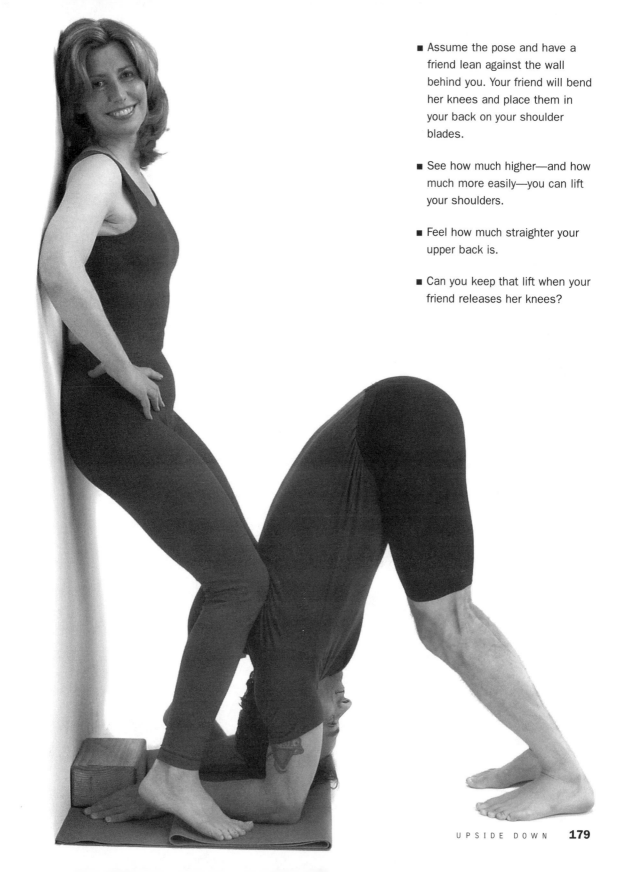

- Assume the pose and have a friend lean against the wall behind you. Your friend will bend her knees and place them in your back on your shoulder blades.

- See how much higher—and how much more easily—you can lift your shoulders.

- Feel how much straighter your upper back is.

- Can you keep that lift when your friend releases her knees?

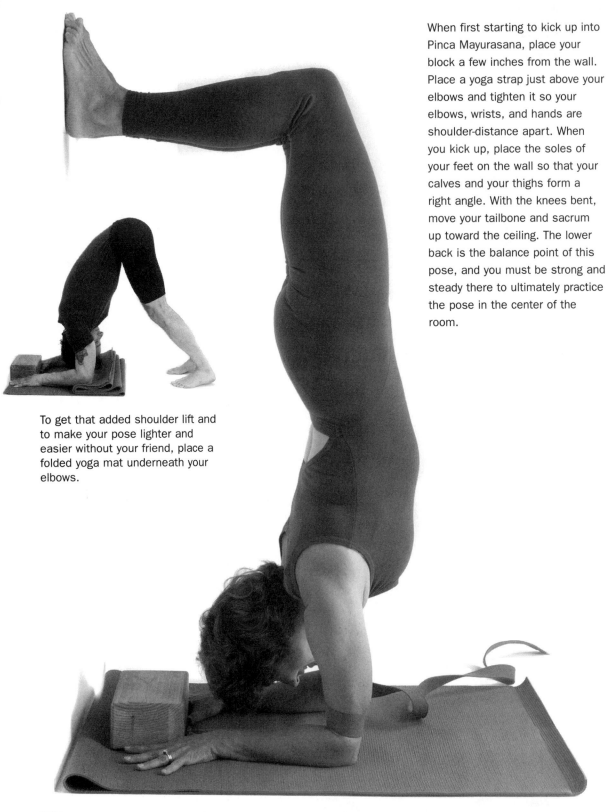

When first starting to kick up into Pinca Mayurasana, place your block a few inches from the wall. Place a yoga strap just above your elbows and tighten it so your elbows, wrists, and hands are shoulder-distance apart. When you kick up, place the soles of your feet on the wall so that your calves and your thighs form a right angle. With the knees bent, move your tailbone and sacrum up toward the ceiling. The lower back is the balance point of this pose, and you must be strong and steady there to ultimately practice the pose in the center of the room.

To get that added shoulder lift and to make your pose lighter and easier without your friend, place a folded yoga mat underneath your elbows.

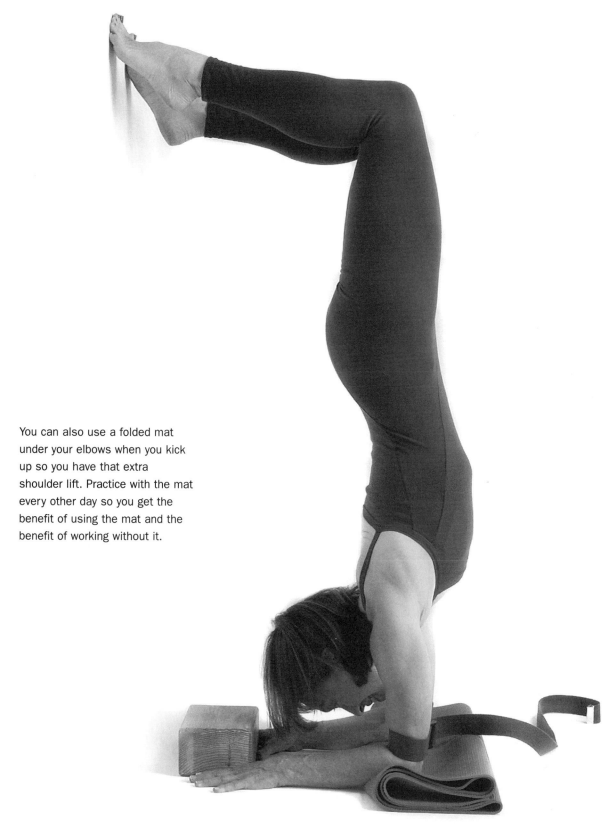

You can also use a folded mat under your elbows when you kick up so you have that extra shoulder lift. Practice with the mat every other day so you get the benefit of using the mat and the benefit of working without it.

SIRSASANA
Headstand

Sirsasana is called the king of all poses. In his classic book, *Light on Yoga* (Schocken Books, 1966), the internationally renowned yoga master B.K.S. Iyengar tells us why.

> The skull encases the brain, which controls the nervous system and the organs of sense. The brain is the seat of intelligence, knowledge, discrimination, wisdom, and power. It is the seat of Brahman, the soul. A country cannot prosper without a proper king or constitutional head to guide it; so also the human body cannot prosper without a healthy brain. . . . Regular practice of Sirsasana makes healthy pure blood flow through the brain cells. This rejuvenates them so that thinking power increases and thoughts become clearer. The asana is a tonic for those who tire easily. It ensures a proper blood supply to the pituitary and pineal glands in the brain. Our growth, health, and vitality depend on the proper functioning of these two glands. . . . Regular and precise practice of Sirsasana develops the body, disciplines the mind, and widens the horizons of the spirit.

- Fold a blanket and kneel down in front of it.

- Interlock your fingers so your hands form a "round basket" with the heels of your hands approximately five inches apart.

- Place your hands on the blanket, little-finger-side down. Place the sides of your forearms, shoulder-distance apart, on the blanket.

- Place the crown of your head on the blanket, with the back of your head touching your hands. (See page 189 for a variation.)

- Straighten your knees, come up on your toes, and walk in toward your head until your torso is perpendicular to the floor.

- Press your forearms evenly— from the wrist to the elbow— into the floor.

- Roll the outside edges of your armpits and deltoid muscles forward.

- Lift your shoulders toward the ceiling and keep them lifted throughout the pose.

- Those new to Headstand can kick up one leg at a time. Intermediate and advanced students can bring both legs up at once.

- Stretch the torso evenly toward the ceiling.

- Engage your quadriceps, roll your thighs inward, and stretch your inner and outer thighs toward the ceiling.

- Move the fronts of your thighs toward the backs of your thighs.

- Lift your tailbone and sacrum up toward the ceiling and bring them into the body.

- Firm your hips and bring them into the body.

- Stretch the four corners of your feet toward the ceiling. (See page 13.)

- Stay in the pose as long as you like. Release by bringing both legs down together. Beginners bring one leg down at a time as per page 168. Rest in Child's Pose for a few minutes.

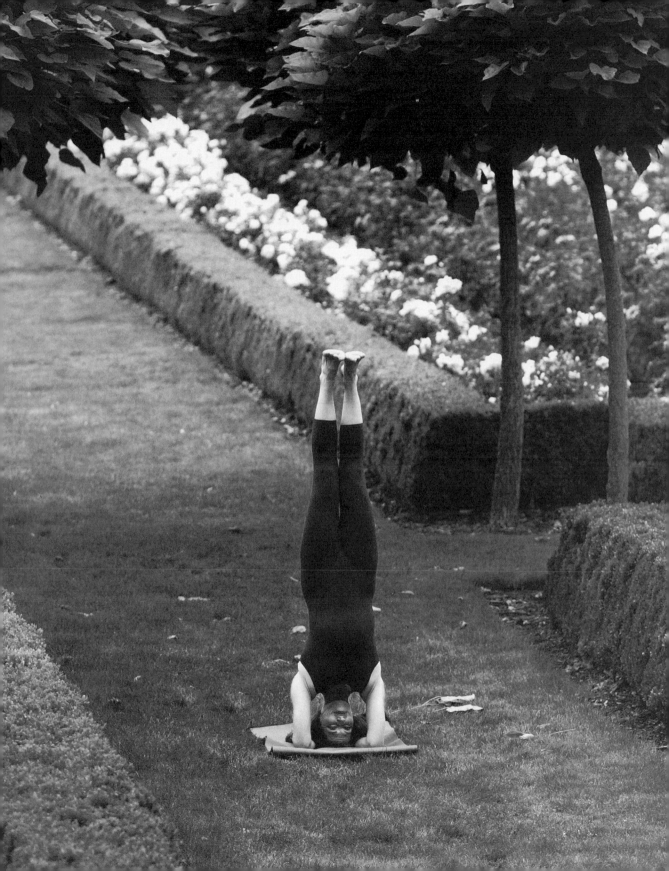

The practice of other poses prepares us for Sirsasana. Yet, even when we think we are ready for Headstand, we often find that we don't have the upper body strength to lift ourselves up or the flexibility to maintain a perpendicular stance. To increase upper body strength, practice Pre-Headstand (see below), Plank (pages 240 and 242), Chaturanga (pages 240 and 242), and the other inversions in this chapter.

For enhancing your flexibility, practice some of the poses described in "Super Stretches" and "Befriending Back Bends." Additionally, here are some tricks that can enhance your Headstand practice.

PRE-HEADSTAND POSES

This pose is similar to Pre—Forearm Balance. Here, however, interlock your fingers so your hands form a "basket" and place the sides of your forearms on the floor. Lift your shoulders as much as you can—or try the friend-as-helper trick or the mat-under-the-elbows trick.

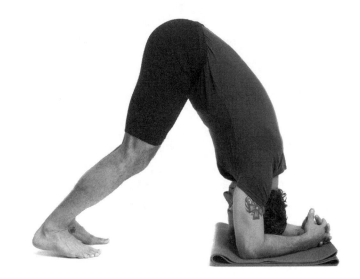

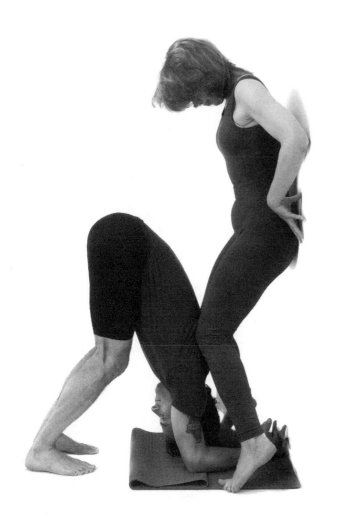

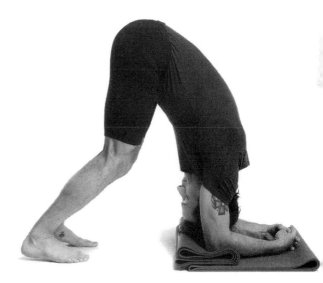

FULL-HEADSTAND TRICKS

The standard way for beginners to practice Headstand is to perform the posture against a wall or in a corner. These techniques are very good, but you have probably seen them in other books. Here are some alternatives to try.

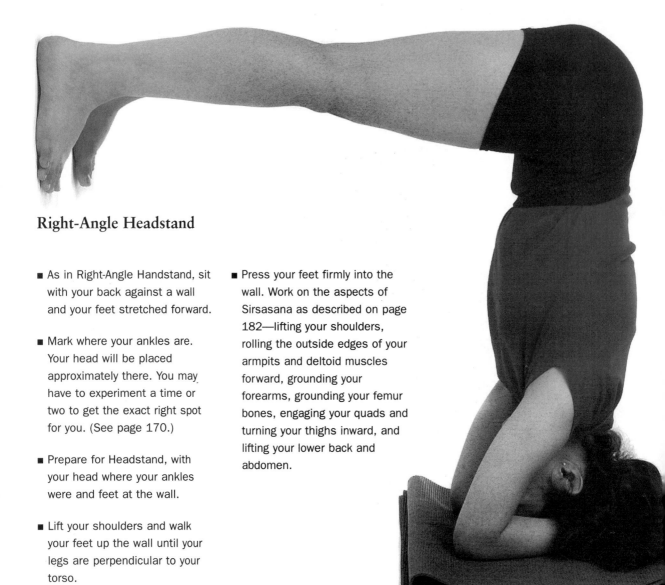

Right-Angle Headstand

- As in Right-Angle Handstand, sit with your back against a wall and your feet stretched forward.

- Mark where your ankles are. Your head will be placed approximately there. You may have to experiment a time or two to get the exact right spot for you. (See page 170.)

- Prepare for Headstand, with your head where your ankles were and feet at the wall.

- Lift your shoulders and walk your feet up the wall until your legs are perpendicular to your torso.

- Press your feet firmly into the wall. Work on the aspects of Sirsasana as described on page 182—lifting your shoulders, rolling the outside edges of your armpits and deltoid muscles forward, grounding your forearms, grounding your femur bones, engaging your quads and turning your thighs inward, and lifting your lower back and abdomen.

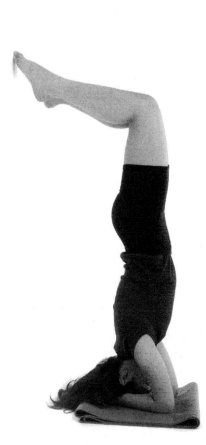

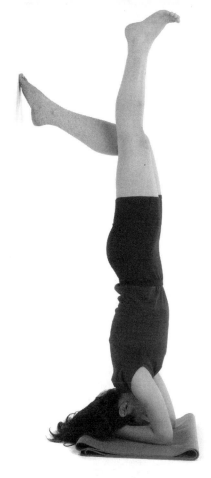

- For this trick, prepare for Headstand with your blanket set up approximately eighteen inches from a wall.

- Come into Headstand and place the balls of your feet on the wall.

- Go through your mental checklist of what you need to do:

  - lift your shoulders

  - roll the outside edges of your armpits and deltoid muscles forward

  - firmly and evenly press your forearms into the floor

  - lengthen your spine and stretch your torso toward the ceiling

  - roll your thighs inward

- Lift the balls of your feet off the wall and press your toes into the wall. By doing so your tailbone and lower back will move up toward the ceiling and into your body. Hold this position firmly.

- When you feel ready, lift one leg over your head and continue to stretch both sides of the spine evenly. Return that foot to the wall, reestablish your toes and

tailbone, and lift the other leg. Allow the trick to teach your body how to work the lower back, and your body will remember.

- When appropriate for you, establish the lift of your lower back and lift both legs overhead.

- Stay in the pose as long as you like. Release and rest in Child's Pose.

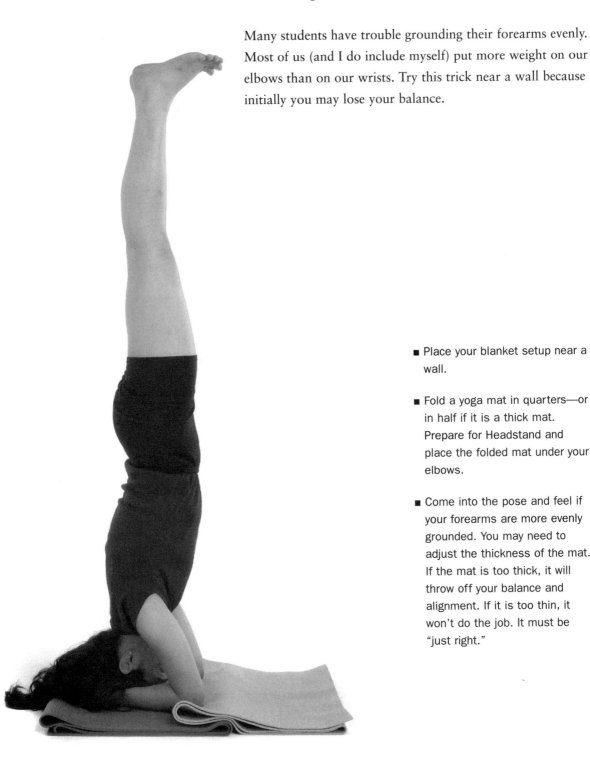

Grounding the Forearms

Many students have trouble grounding their forearms evenly. Most of us (and I do include myself) put more weight on our elbows than on our wrists. Try this trick near a wall because initially you may lose your balance.

- Place your blanket setup near a wall.

- Fold a yoga mat in quarters—or in half if it is a thick mat. Prepare for Headstand and place the folded mat under your elbows.

- Come into the pose and feel if your forearms are more evenly grounded. You may need to adjust the thickness of the mat. If the mat is too thick, it will throw off your balance and alignment. If it is too thin, it won't do the job. It must be "just right."

Trifold Headstand

Many students have difficulty balancing on the crown of their head. For some, their neck hurts; for others, something just feels off. Many, without even realizing it, adjust their head position so they are balancing on a spot that is closer to their forehead.

I was one of those students who had trouble balancing on the crown of my head. My neck hurt and I assumed I would injure myself if I continued in that mode, so I quit practicing Headstand for several months. When I discussed this problem with my friend and teacher, Nancy, she suggested the following trick, which is therapeutic for those with straighter-than-normal cervical spines.

- Fold a towel, thin blanket, or thin yoga mat in half. Then fold it in thirds lengthwise.

- Center the prop on your folded yoga mat and prepare for Headstand.

- Place the part of your head that is about one inch forward of the crown on the prop and come up into Headstand.

- Be near a wall when you first practice this version of Headstand in case you falter.

- Experiment with the placement of your head to find the spot that is most comfortable for you. Consult with a teacher who is trained in yoga therapy if you are still unsure about the placement of your head. It is better to err on the side of caution by not practicing Headstand than to do this pose incorrectly.

SALAMBA SARVANGASANA

Shoulder Stand

B.K.S. Iyengar says that Sarvangasana is the mother of all asanas. "As a mother strives for harmony and happiness in the home, so this asana strives for the harmony and happiness in the human system. It is a panacea for most common ailments." Sarvangasana enhances proper functioning of the body's internal systems, including the glandular, hormonal, respiratory, digestive, circulatory, reproductive, and nervous systems. "It is one of the greatest boons conferred on humanity by our ancient sages."*

Some schools of yoga teach the practice of Shoulder Stand on the floor. When I do Shoulder Stand on the floor my neck feels constricted and my upper back feels unnaturally curved. Using blankets under the shoulders, which is recommended in the Iyengar tradition, gives me more freedom in my neck and my back feels straighter. If you are unaccustomed to using blankets, try the blankets a few times and see if you feel more freedom in your Shoulder Stand.

I also recommend using a strap around the upper arms, just above the elbows, which keeps the arms from splaying outward while in the pose. Before you go into the pose, prepare the strap by making a loop that is shoulder-distance wide. You will put it on as you are preparing to go into the posture.

- Arrange two to five firm blankets on the floor. Make sure that the smooth, folded edges of the blankets are aligned. That is where your neck will be. Place a folded yoga mat on top of the blankets.

- Lie with your shoulders, neck, and arms on the blanket/yoga mat setup. Your head will be off of the blankets and your shoulders will be on the smooth, folded edge.

- Beginners can perform the pose as described on the following pages.

- Intermediate students can first come into Plow Pose.

- Place a looped yoga strap around arms, just above your elbows.

- Make sure the loop is shoulder-distance in length.

- Clasp your hands, roll your shoulders under, and then place your palms on your back so that the heel of your hands will be at the bottoms of your shoulder blades.

- Bring your legs overhead, one at a time.

- Stretch your entire body upward—from your armpits to your toes.

- Engage your quadriceps, roll your thighs inward, and press the fronts of your thighs toward the backs of your thighs.

- Lift your tailbone and lower back toward the ceiling and bring them deep into your body.

- Firm your hips and bring them in toward your body.

- Widen the tops of your shoulders outward, from your neck to the edges of your shoulders.

- Soften your throat and bring your chin to your chest.

- To lift yourself more in the pose, walk your hands down your back (toward your shoulders) and lift yourself higher.

- To release, come into Halasana (Plow), and then roll out.

- Lie on the blankets or on the floor to rest for a few minutes.

*B.K.S. Iyengar, *Light on Yoga*, Schocken Books, 1966.

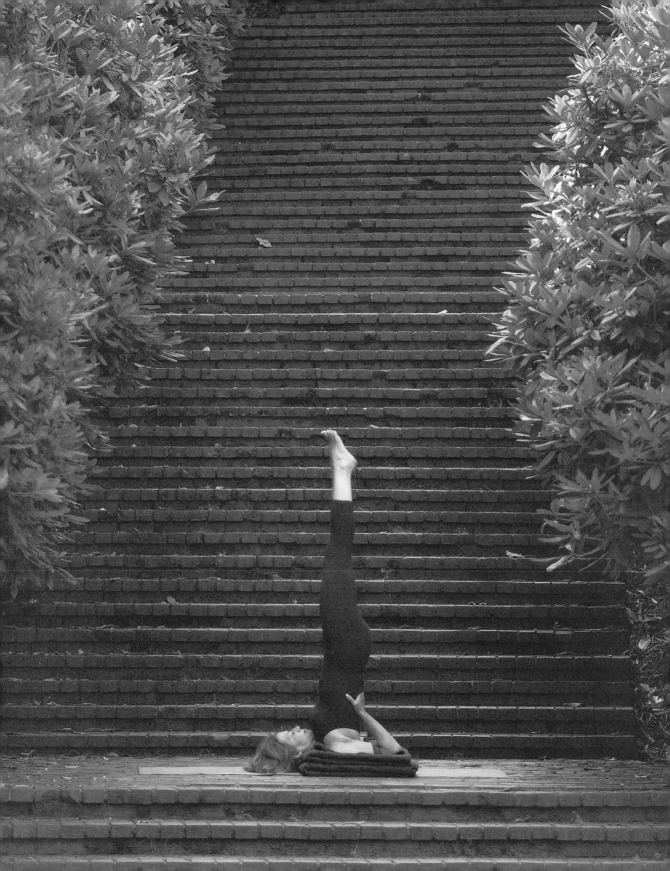

Like a good mother, Sarvangasana at times will coddle you and at other times will challenge you to your greatest abilities. However, the benefits of Salamba Sarvangasana far outweigh the challenges that accompany mastering it.

In the early phases of learning Shoulder Stand, many of us struggle with keeping our chest open, keeping our throats soft, and keeping the lift of our legs and torso. Initially we often feel exhausted and frustrated instead of nourished, relaxed, and refreshed. If you can consciously drop the struggle and continue with your efforts to master the pose, you will find much more rest in Shoulder Stand. These tricks will help.

True Beginner Shoulder Stand

When you are first learning the pose, try using a chair in this manner:

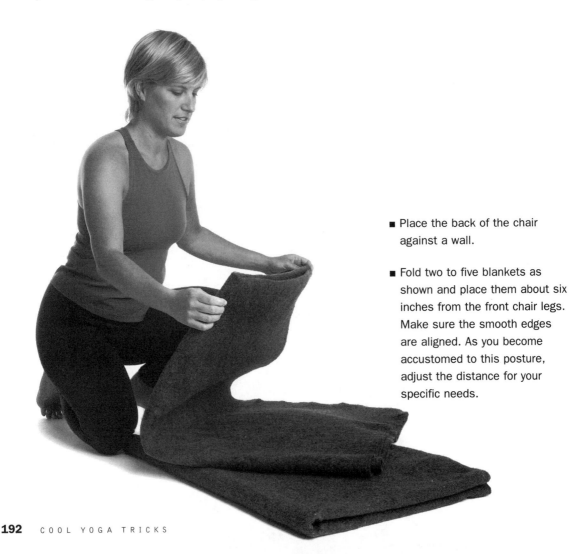

- Place the back of the chair against a wall.

- Fold two to five blankets as shown and place them about six inches from the front chair legs. Make sure the smooth edges are aligned. As you become accustomed to this posture, adjust the distance for your specific needs.

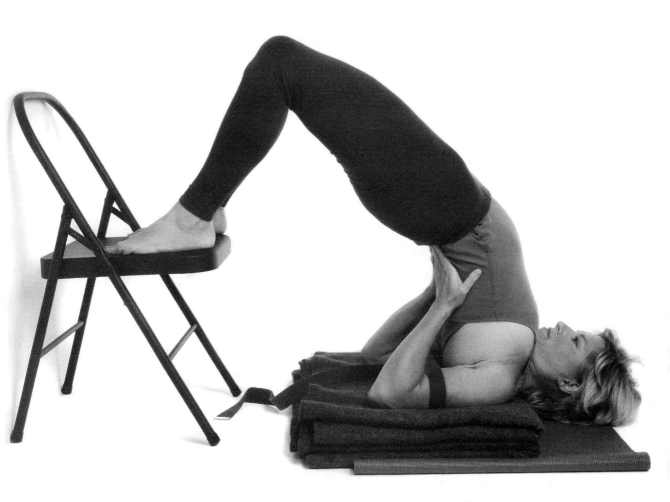

- Lie down on the blankets so your torso and neck are on the blankets and your head is off the blankets. Your feet are on the chair seat.

- Clasp the front chair legs.

- Place the soles of your feet on the chair seat and lift your hips.

- Roll your shoulders under, and firmly ground your arms into the blankets.

- Lift your hips to your absolute maximum and lift the backs of your thighs toward the fronts of your thighs. Roll your thighs inward.

- Move your tailbone toward your knees and into your body.

- Raise the back of your torso toward the front of your torso and lift your chest toward the ceiling.

- Widen the tops of your shoulders outward, from your neck to the edge of your shoulders.

- Soften your throat and bring your chest toward your chin.

- When you first start to practice this posture, hold the pose for a minute or two. It is best to do the pose properly—without slumping your chest, hips, and legs—for a short time than to practice the posture improperly for a longer period of time.

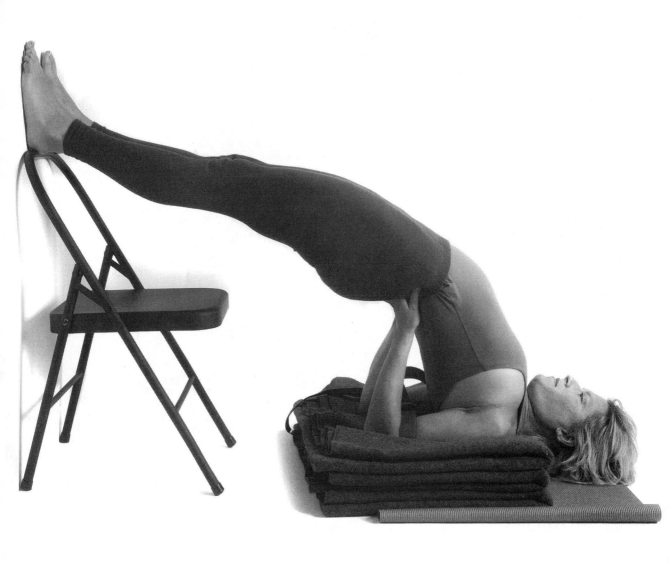

■ As an alternative posture, bring
the soles of your feet to the
wall and your heels to the top of
the chair. Continue to work the
legs, hips, and lower back.

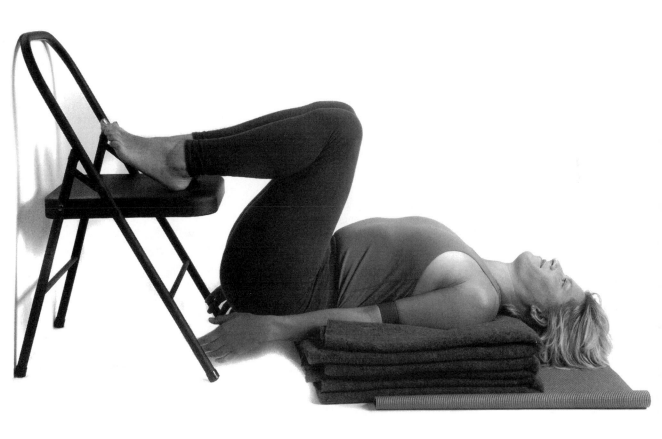

■ After releasing, rest with your
feet on the chair seat for a few
minutes.

Second-Stage Beginner Shoulder Stand

After practicing the previous pose for several weeks and feeling comfortable in it, you are ready to move on to Stage Two.

- Place your folded blanket setup approximately fifteen inches from the wall. Adjust accordingly for your height. Have a chair about two feet behind your blankets.

- Lie down on the blankets with your torso, shoulders, and neck on the blankets and your head off the blankets. Bend your knees and walk your feet up the wall.

- Lift your hips and move them toward your head.

- Place a strap that is shoulder-distance wide around your upper arms near your elbows.

- Clasp your hands and roll your shoulders under. Place your palms on your back—with the heels of your palms at the bottoms of your shoulder blades—and press firmly.

- Firm the hips and move them inward. Move your tailbone toward your knees and into your body.

- Roll your thighs inward and stretch your inner thighs upward toward the ceiling.

- Bring the back of your torso toward the front of your torso. Expand your chest.

- Widen the tops of your shoulders outward, from your neck to the edges of your shoulders.

- Soften your throat and move your chest toward your chin.

- Stay in the pose as long as you like. Release by coming into plow pose and rolling out. Rest on the floor or on your blankets for a few minutes.

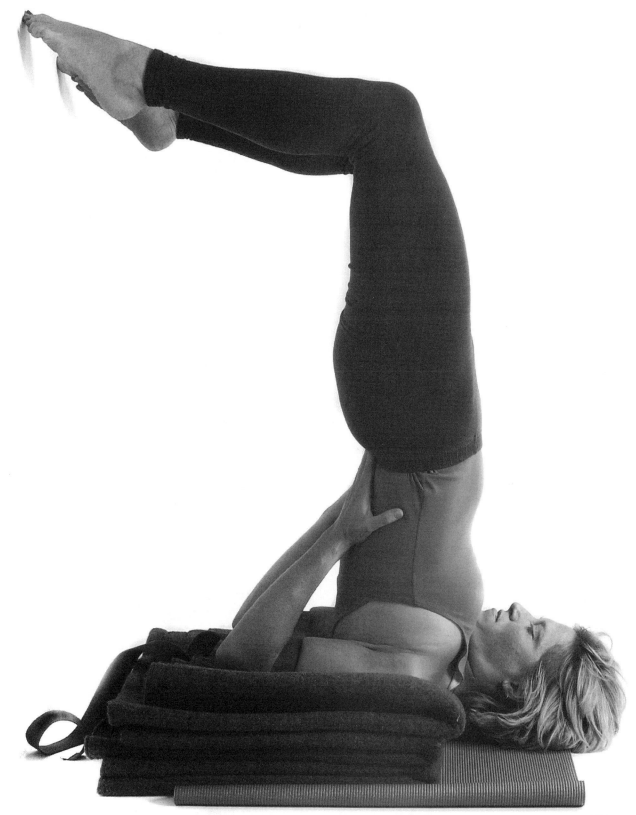

- When you are ready to try balancing with all of your alignment techniques in place, lift one leg straight over your body. Adjust yourself again. Then bring the other foot to join it. Adjust yourself again.

- Look at your heart and breathe calmly and evenly.

- If at any point you feel as though you are collapsing, bring your toes back to the chair (Half Halasana or Plow). Press your toes firmly into the chair seat, which helps you lift your spine and firm your legs. Then go back into Full Shoulder Stand, one leg at a time. You can do this several times per session.

- Release by gently rolling down from Half Halasana.

- Adjust yourself so your head is on the blankets and rest for a few minutes.

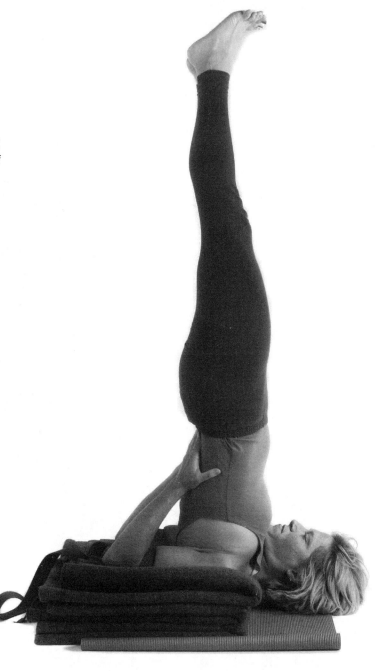

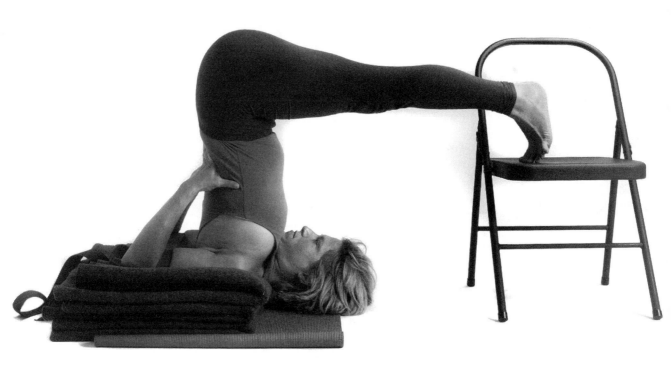

Supported Shoulder Stand and Plow

If Shoulder Stand is the mother, this is when she pampers you the most. This is my absolute favorite combination of asanas. I get so relaxed that I often fall asleep.

The first couple of times you try this posture, have a friend help you. Specifically, have him hold the chair for you to ensure that it won't topple over. If no one is around to help you, place the chair at the wall. After you've tried this pose a couple of times, you will get the hang of it and be able to get in and out of it easily. But be sure to have a sturdy chair. If you are using a metal folding chair, use a heavy, high-quality one rather than a lighter-weight one. Once you are comfortable getting in and out of the pose, you can place the chair in the middle of the room if you prefer, and you can add a bolster for more comfort.

You will need one to three sturdy blankets for these poses. Fold the blankets in quarters, and then into thirds. Place the folded, smooth edges of the blankets away from the chair legs. This is where your shoulders will rest. You will need to experiment with the height of the blankets. One blanket too many or too few can make a huge difference in how you feel in this pose. So experiment with the number of blankets you use; the results are well worth the effort.

You will need a second chair placed behind the blankets for Supported Plow. While I highly recommend using a Halasana bench for this pose, they are a little costly. Practice using a chair as pictured here. Those who are tall may want to place some folded blankets on the chair seat to increase its height.

Make sure the smooth edges are aligned.

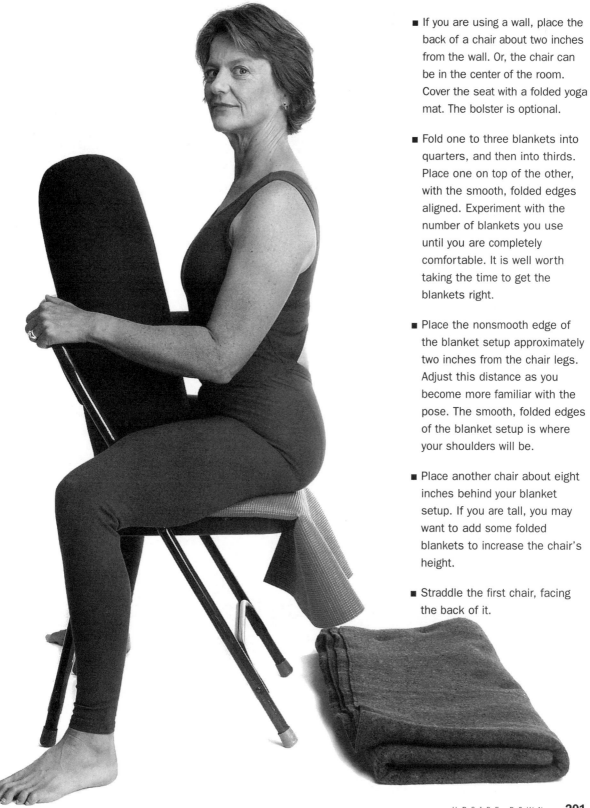

- If you are using a wall, place the back of a chair about two inches from the wall. Or, the chair can be in the center of the room. Cover the seat with a folded yoga mat. The bolster is optional.

- Fold one to three blankets into quarters, and then into thirds. Place one on top of the other, with the smooth, folded edges aligned. Experiment with the number of blankets you use until you are completely comfortable. It is well worth taking the time to get the blankets right.

- Place the nonsmooth edge of the blanket setup approximately two inches from the chair legs. Adjust this distance as you become more familiar with the pose. The smooth, folded edges of the blanket setup is where your shoulders will be.

- Place another chair about eight inches behind your blanket setup. If you are tall, you may want to add some folded blankets to increase the chair's height.

- Straddle the first chair, facing the back of it.

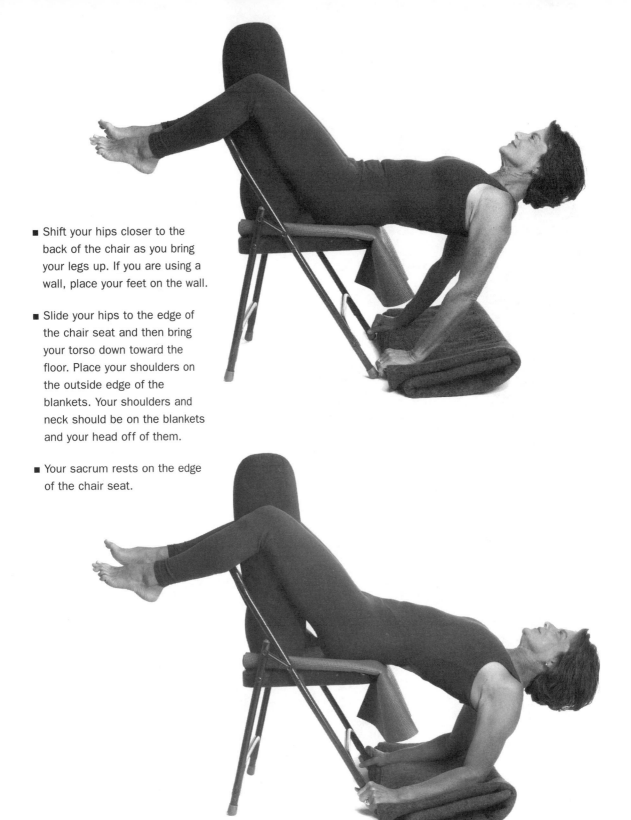

- Shift your hips closer to the back of the chair as you bring your legs up. If you are using a wall, place your feet on the wall.

- Slide your hips to the edge of the chair seat and then bring your torso down toward the floor. Place your shoulders on the outside edge of the blankets. Your shoulders and neck should be on the blankets and your head off of them.

- Your sacrum rests on the edge of the chair seat.

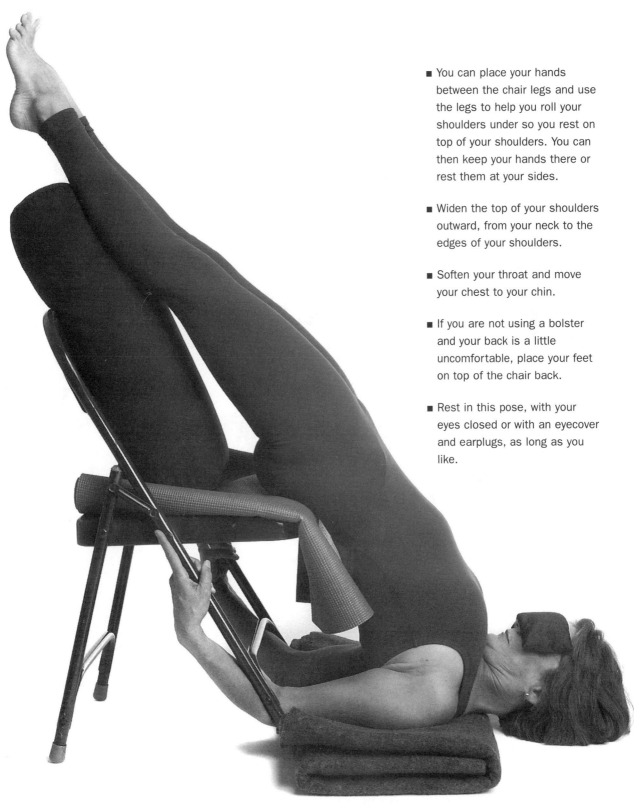

- You can place your hands between the chair legs and use the legs to help you roll your shoulders under so you rest on top of your shoulders. You can then keep your hands there or rest them at your sides.

- Widen the top of your shoulders outward, from your neck to the edges of your shoulders.

- Soften your throat and move your chest to your chin.

- If you are not using a bolster and your back is a little uncomfortable, place your feet on top of the chair back.

- Rest in this pose, with your eyes closed or with an eyecover and earplugs, as long as you like.

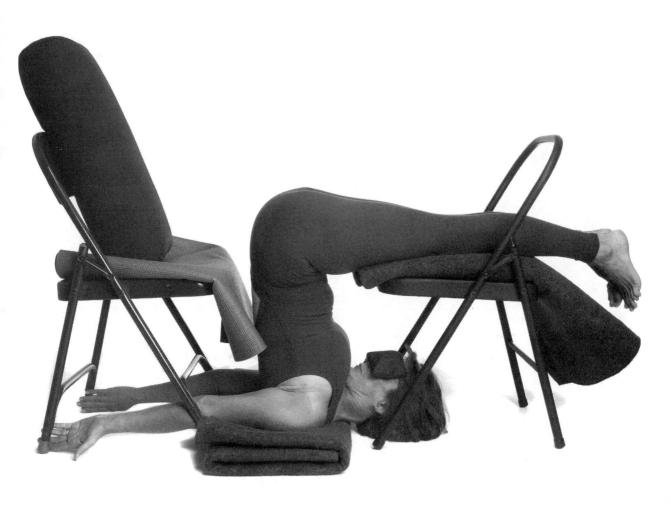

When you are ready, lift your
sacrum off the chair and bring
your thighs to the chair behind
you. Rest as long as you like. To
release, go back into Supported
Shoulder Stand and slide your
hips to the blankets.

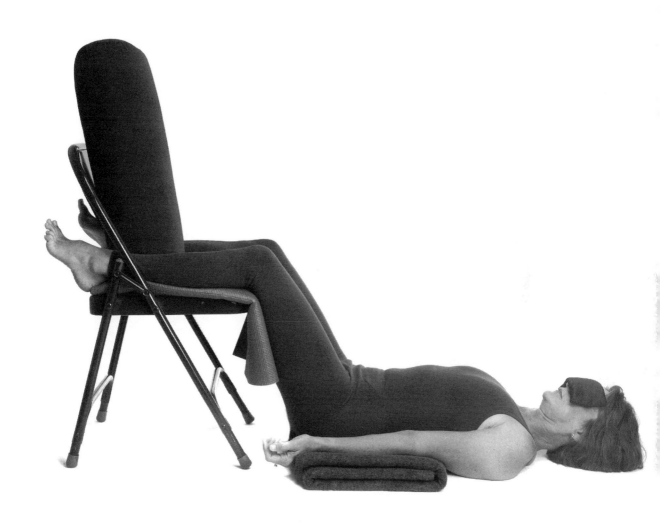

Rest for a few minutes with your
legs on the chair seat before
getting up.

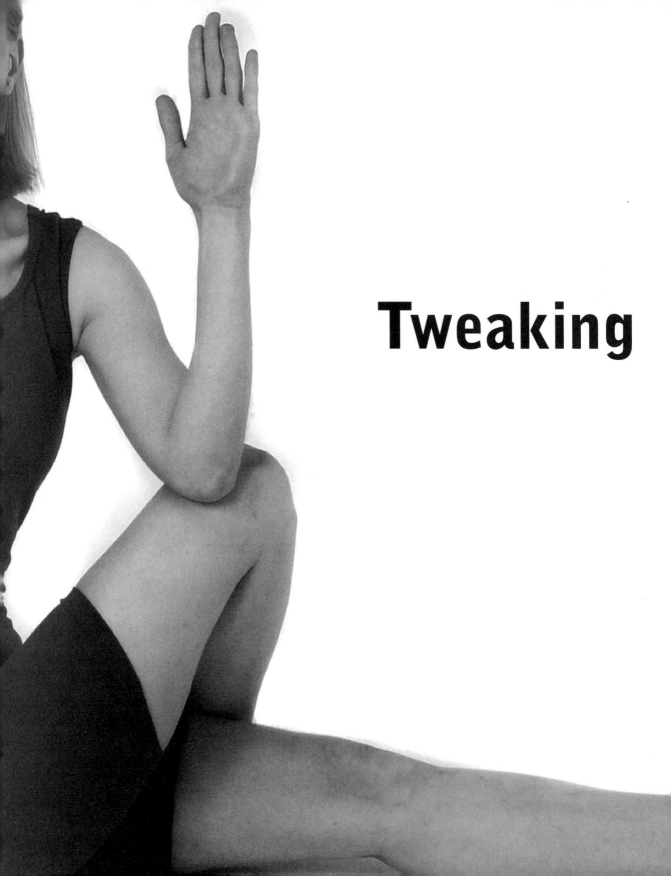

Tweaking

*We often need to twist in our everyday lives. Active,
deliberate twisting, as we do in our yoga practice,
keeps us flexible in different ways than those achieved
in stretching and strengthening exercises.*

Your Twists

Twists activate the spine, the surrounding muscles, and the internal organs. They improve circulation to the vertebrae and to the internal organs. Lengthening and stretching the spine through a practice of twists counteracts the normal effects of gravity, which compress our spine.

It is important to have a strong base from which you twist your spine. In seated twists, the hips, legs, feet, and often the hands form the base. In standing twists, the feet must be firmly planted on the floor and the legs must be very firm, as they form the base of the twists. It is of great importance to twist from the base or very lowest part of the spine. A firm, strong base allows this action to occur more readily.

Prior to practicing twists, you should perform a few forward bends so that your back muscles are warmed up and can more readily receive the twisting action. If you are practicing twists after your back bend practice, practice only gentle twists.

As a general rule, you should enter into twists carefully and deepen the twists gradually. In seated twists, sitting on a blanket helps lift your spine, as extending your spine can become increasingly difficult as you deepen the twists.

PARIVRTTA TRIKONASANA
Revolved Triangle Pose

Parivrtta Trikonasana is a graceful posture that enhances strength, flexibility, and balance.

- Stand with your feet three and a half to four feet apart with your arms outstretched.

- Turn your right foot out ninety degrees and your left foot toward your right by about sixty degrees.

- Align the heel of your forward foot with the arch of your back foot.

- Rotate your torso to the right until the front of your torso completely faces your forward leg.

- Lift your quadriceps. Rotate your right thigh outward and your left thigh inward.

- Press your back heel firmly into the ground and keep it strongly grounded throughout the pose.

- Rotate your torso to the right while extending your right arm and torso forward.

- Place your palm or fist on the side of your right foot.

- Be sure that your torso is aligned with your hips.

- Bring the right hip back and the left hip forward.

- Continue to lift your quads and rotate your thighs toward each other.

- Bring the fronts of your thighs to the backs of your thighs (in other words, ground your femur bones).

- Stretch your left hand from your shoulder to the floor and press your hand firmly into the floor.

- Bring your right hand up, aligned with your shoulder. Stretch that arm from the shoulder to the fingertips. Turn your head and gaze at your hand.

- On your inhalation, lengthen your spine. On your exhalation, twist farther toward the right from the very bottom of your spine.

- Unwind on an inhalation and repeat on the other side.

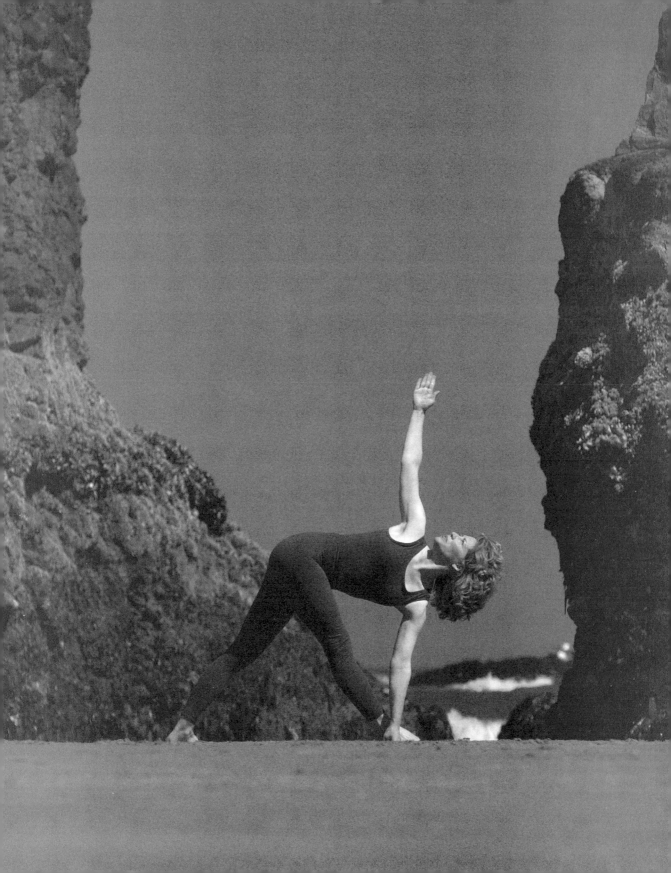

Of the many challenges of Parivrtta Trikonasana, among the most difficult are keeping the back heel pressed firmly into the floor, bringing the front hipbone backward, bringing the back hipbone forward, and placing your hand on the floor. These challenges result from tight hips. Yet proper actions are of utmost importance to experience the benefits of this posture.

Twisting-in-Trikonasana Tricks

These tricks will help you overcome all of these challenges, even if your hips are tight. As in all twisting poses, the stronger the base, the more easily the spine will twist—and from the lowest point on the spine. The grounded back heel is the foundation of this posture's base. If your back heel does not firmly press into the floor—and if your hand doesn't touch the floor—these tricks are for you.

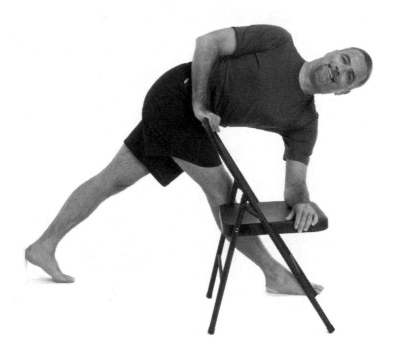

- Prepare for Revolved Triangle by placing your back heel against a wall with your feet three and a half to four feet apart. Have some props handy.

- Come into Revolved Triangle as described on page 208, and

place your forearm on the chair seat.

- The arm that should be over your head is on the back of the chair. With the aid of the chair, twist your spine toward the chair. Be careful that you keep

your torso over your hips, as it is easy to lean toward the chair in this pose.

- Continually press your heel firmly into the wall.

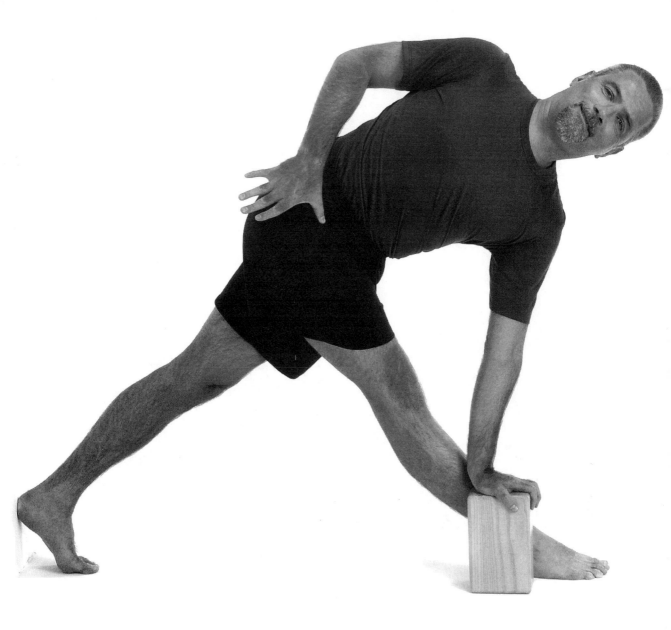

- As you progress in your practice
  of Parivrtta Trikonasana, place
  your forward hand on a block.

- To help press the forward hip
  backward, place your thumb in
  your hip crease and push your
  hip and femur bone backward.
  This will help enhance the twist.

Or you can have a friend help you
roll your thighs and bring your
front hipbone back.

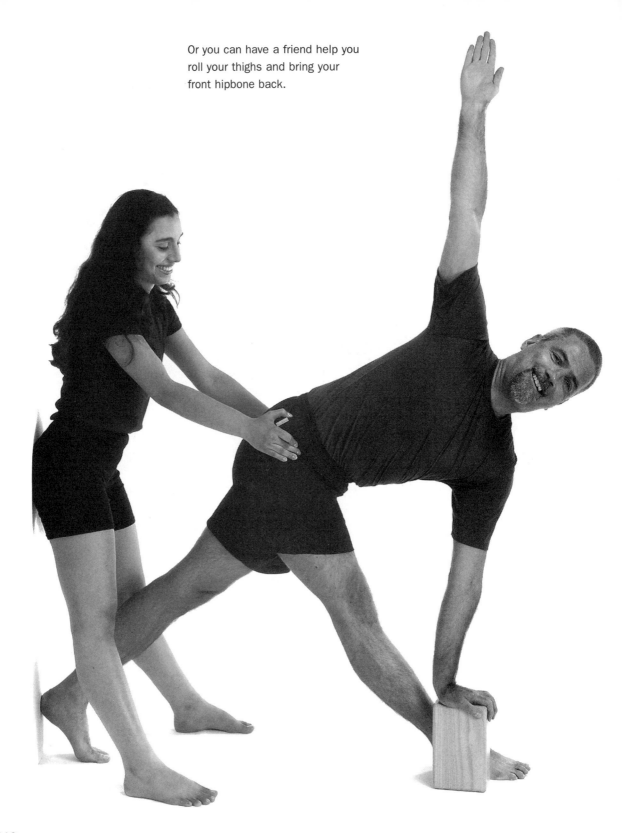

Another option for thigh rolling is to place a strap around your forward thigh (see instructions on page 88) and rotate your thigh outward by pulling on the strap as you enter the pose. You can release the strap when you feel that your hip is adequately back and your thigh and spine properly rotated.

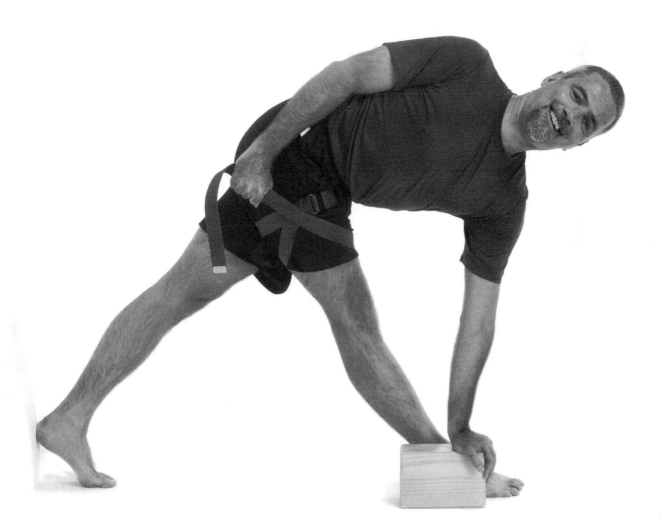

Downward Dog to Revolved Triangle

An easy way to practice Revolved Triangle is to enter it from Downward Dog. The directions are for those who need their heel at the wall and a block for their hand. As you progress in your practice of this pose, you can try this with your hands and feet on the floor.

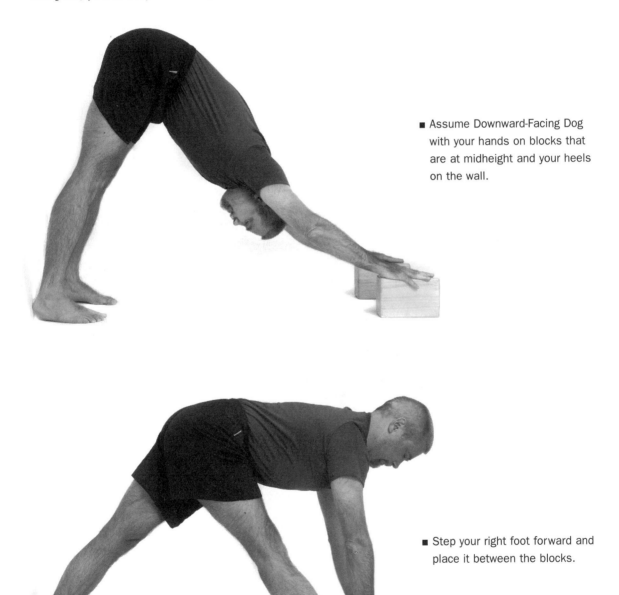

- Assume Downward-Facing Dog with your hands on blocks that are at midheight and your heels on the wall.

- Step your right foot forward and place it between the blocks.

- Bring your right front hipbone backward and the left hipbone forward. Twist toward the right from the very lowest area of your spine. You may need to bring your block closer to your ankle.

- Rotate your torso to face the right and place your left hand on the block.

- Make the alignment adjustments suggested on page 208.

- Release, come back to Downward Dog, and repeat with your left leg forward.

- As you gain proficiency, you will no longer need the blocks. But don't give up the blocks too quickly and risk performing the pose improperly without them.

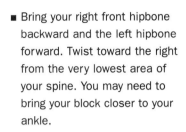

Revolving the Torso

In this trick, you will practice grounding your back heel on a folded mat and using the wall to rotate your torso.

■ Assume the Pre-Revolved Triangle position facing the wall and with your back heel on a folded mat.

■ Come into the pose.

■ Place your forward hand on the floor or on a block and your other hand on the wall.

■ Use the leverage of your hand on the wall to rotate your torso.

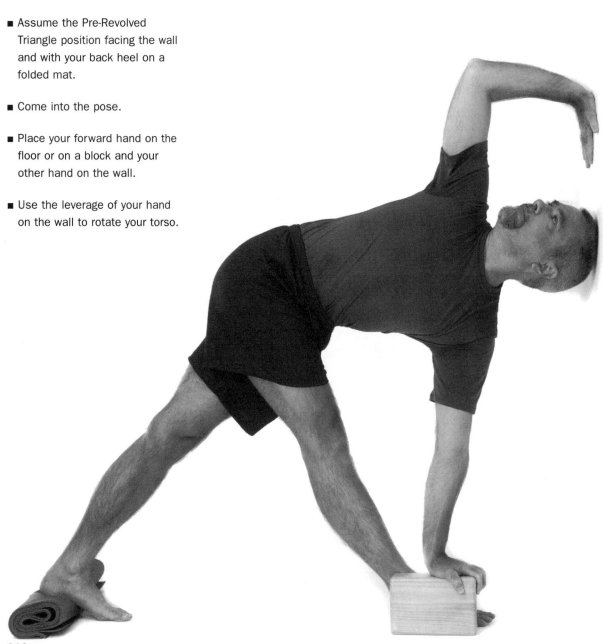

Super-Twisting in Trikonasana

Here's a method of enhancing your twist a great deal. It involves the use of a slant board. If you don't have a slant board, my guess is that a smooth two-by-four will work just as well. Try this trick because it is truly awesome.

This can be done with your hand on either a block or a chair.

- Assume your favorite starting position for Revolved Triangle.

- When your torso is turned forward, place a slant board between your thighs, as high as possible. The flat side of the board should be on the inside of your forward leg. About six inches of the board should be in front of you.

- Hold the front of the slant board with the hand that is on the same side as your forward foot.

- Move into the pose, placing your back hand on the floor or your prop.

- Pull the board in the same direction you are twisting.

- Hold as long as you like. Unwind on an inhalation and repeat on the second side.

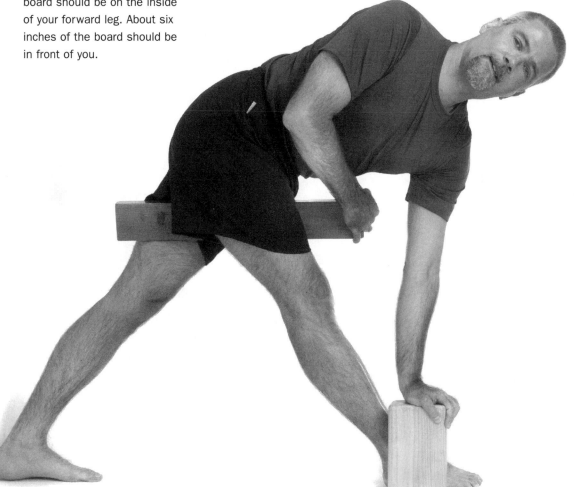

Additional Twisting Tricks

With the understanding that proper grounding of your body is the base of your twist, here are some tricks to help you perform some of the basic twisting poses. Try the ones shown here and see if you can take that understanding into your practice of other twists.

Here are some easy versions of more complicated twists.

- If your torso is long and your arms are short or if you simply want added extension, place your back hand on a block behind you when doing seated twists.

- *Very important:* When performing twists in which the sole of one foot is on the floor, firmly press your foot into the floor. Doing so stabilizes your base and helps you twist from the lowest point of your spine.

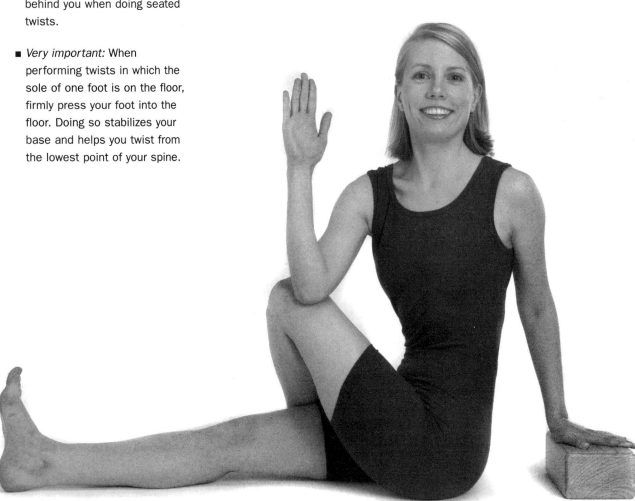

In Pasasana, many students have trouble wrapping their arms around their bodies and pressing their feet firmly into the floor. If you have similar troubles, take your twist to the wall.

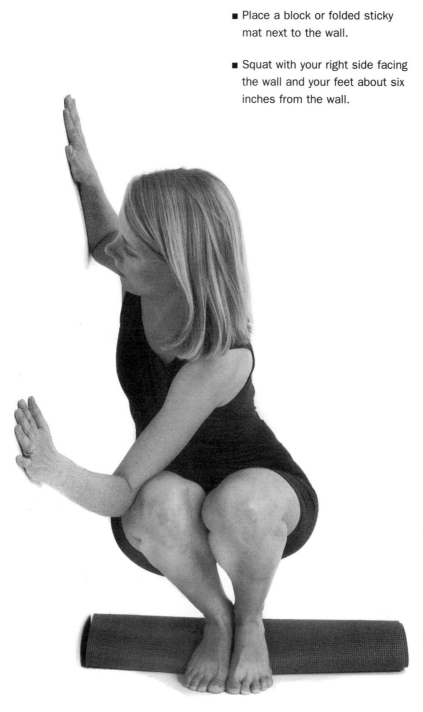

- Place a block or folded sticky mat next to the wall.

- Squat with your right side facing the wall and your feet about six inches from the wall.

- Turn toward the wall, pulling your tummy with you, if necessary.

- Place your left arm, about two inches above your elbow, on the side of your right thigh, near the knee. Then place both hands on the wall.

- Press your heels into the block or yoga mat.

- Press your left arm and right leg into each other.

- Inhale, lift your spine, and relax your shoulders.

- Exhale and twist, from the lowest point of your spine, toward the wall.

- The more you can ground your heels and press the arm and leg into each other, the more your twist will come from the lowest part of your spine.

- Continue the motions of inhaling and lifting the spine, exhaling and twisting the spine, several times. Each time you twist, maintain the level of that twist—that is, do not allow your torso to revert backward.

- Unwind on an inhalation. Switch sides and repeat on the left side.

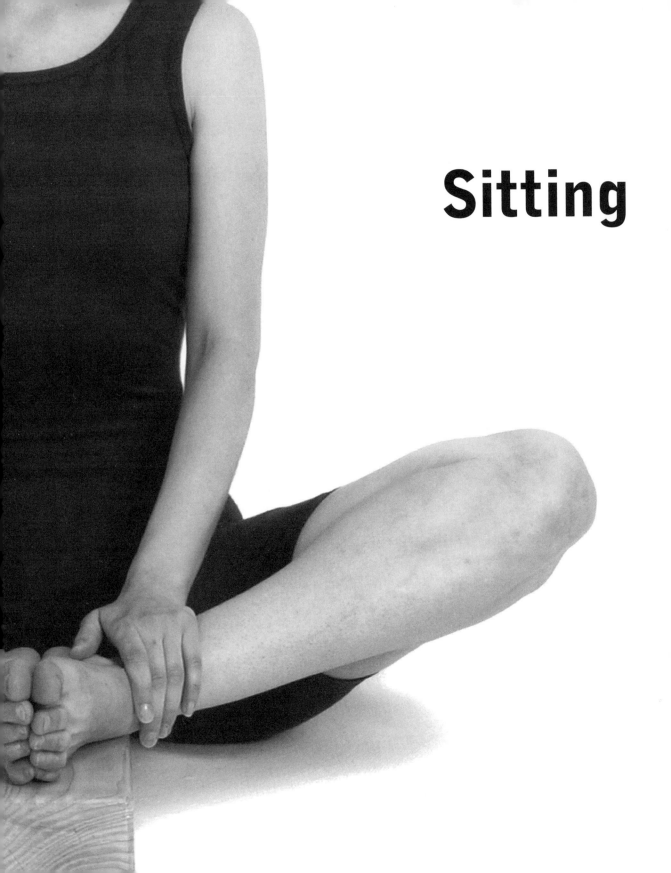

Sitting

Secrets

For those who find sitting in a simple cross-legged position on the floor difficult, you will find yogic seated postures completely forbidding—creating more stress and strain than you ever dreamed possible. Yet as they are mastered, these seated postures increase strength and flexibility in the lower back and flexibility in the hips, thighs, knees, and ankles. Many of the yogic seated poses calm and quiet the nervous system and, ultimately, the mind. That is why they are used for meditation.

In the interest of space, I have included tricks for only two seated postures—Baddha Konasana and Padmasana. I have chosen Baddha Konasana because it is probably the most commonly practiced seated pose. In fact, many people who don't practice yoga do this pose to warm up for running, biking, and other sports. Lotus is included because it is so difficult and so many students want to master it.

BADDHA KONASANA
Bound Angle Pose

Baddha Konasana, Bound Angle Pose, improves circulation and increases flexibility in the legs, hips, abdomen, and lower back. When performed properly, it also strengthens the muscles of the lower back.

This pose is a blessing for women with menstrual problems, and regular practice is recommended during pregnancy.

- Sit erect with your legs extended.

- Place your right hand under your right knee and bring your leg in toward your body.

- Place your right hand around your right ankle and bring your right foot to the middle of your body, with the side of your right foot on the floor.

- Repeat the same movements with your left hand and leg, and place the sole of your left foot so that it joins the sole of your right foot.

- Continually press the soles of your feet together, and extend your inner and outer thighs toward your knees.

- Lift your lower back and lower abdomen up and slightly in toward each other. Lift your sternum and relax your shoulders, throat, and neck.

- Hold your toes or place your hands behind you to help maintain a straight spine.

- Hold the pose as long as you like.

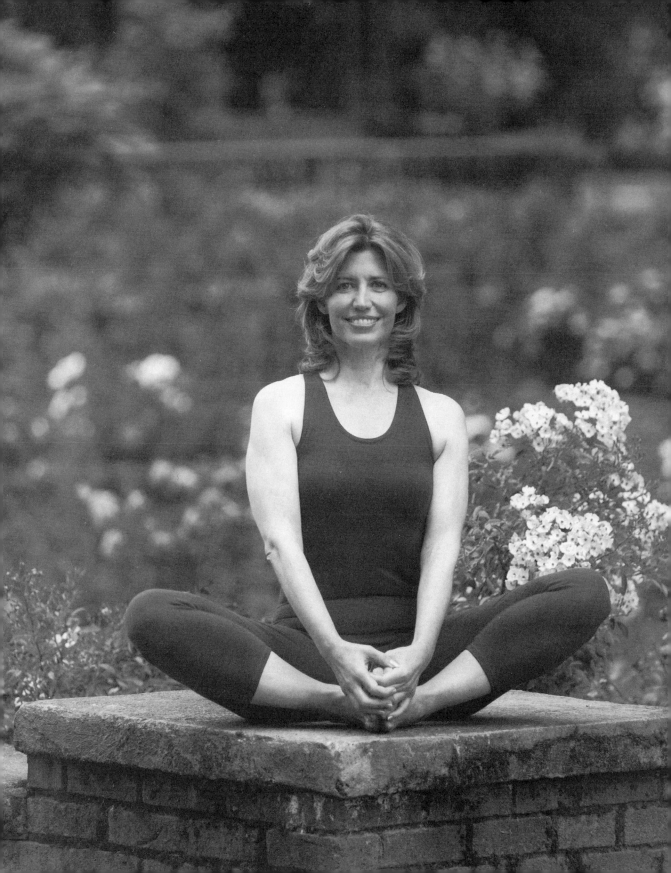

BADDHA KONASANA

The goal of Baddha Konasana is *not* to get your knees to the floor as quickly as possible. Rather, the intent is to lengthen your inner and outer thighs, strengthen your lower back, and increase flexibility in your legs, hips, knees, and back. These benefits may allow your knees to reach the floor, but forcing your knees to the floor could cause harm.

Lack of flexibility prevents many students from sitting in this pose comfortably. But perhaps the most difficult aspect, both for the flexible and the flexibly impaired, is keeping the back straight. This section presents tricks for those whose bodies object to sitting this way, and for students who are looking for new-and-improved ways to enhance their practice of Bound Angle Pose.

For those who are very stiff, sitting in a chair makes this pose doable. Use a strap around your feet and gently pull the strap toward you. This trick keeps your back straight and puts less strain on your hips and knees. As you progress, place your feet on the same chair you are sitting on.

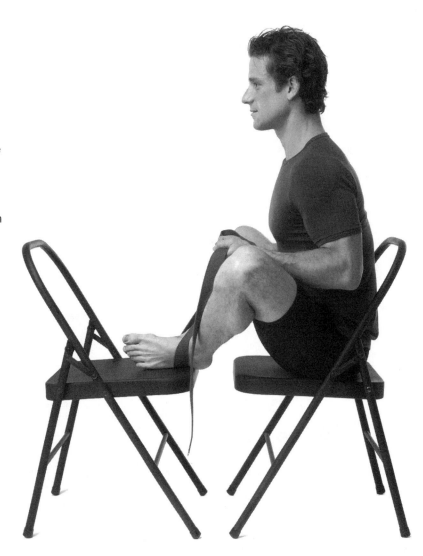

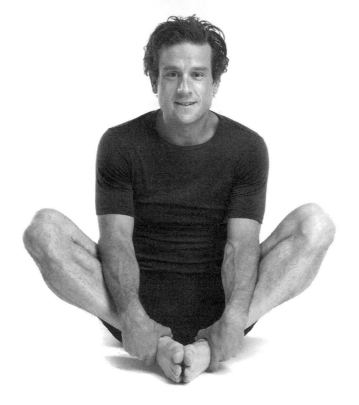

When sitting in Baddha Konasana, if your knees are at or above your waist, as Jimmy's are above, you need to sit on enough blankets so your knees will fall below your waist. Notice how when sitting on blankets his legs come down and his spine lengthens.

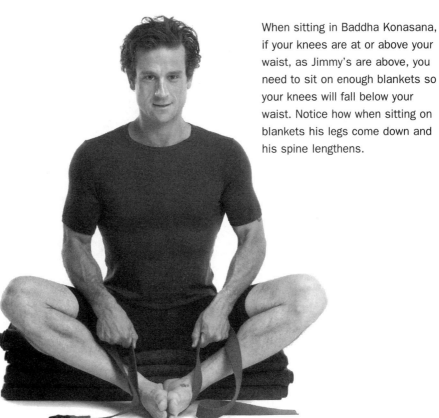

Increasing Flexibility

It is obvious that these tricks increase your inner thigh flexibility. What may come as a surprise is that they also increase the flexibility in your outer hips and lower back.

Sit with your back flush against a wall and come into Baddha Konasana as described on page 222. The wall helps you to keep your back straight and increases the extension in your inner thighs. Then, try these tricks to enhance the extendability of your inner thighs.

■ First, place a block, at its narrowest width, between your feet. Continually press the soles of your feet into the block. It is easier to press your feet into the block than it is to press them into each other.

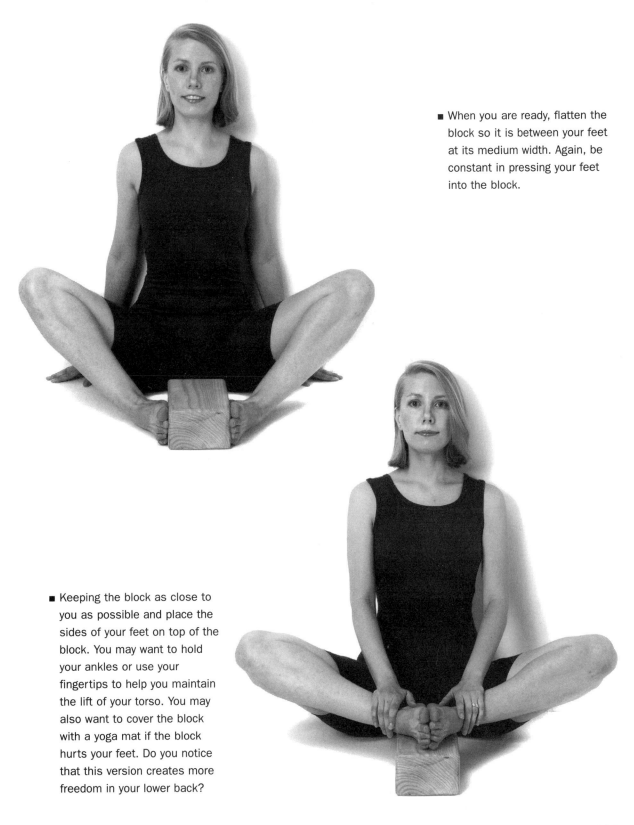

■ When you are ready, flatten the block so it is between your feet at its medium width. Again, be constant in pressing your feet into the block.

■ Keeping the block as close to you as possible and place the sides of your feet on top of the block. You may want to hold your ankles or use your fingertips to help you maintain the lift of your torso. You may also want to cover the block with a yoga mat if the block hurts your feet. Do you notice that this version creates more freedom in your lower back?

Lifting Your Back in Baddha Konasana

Maintaining the lift of the lower back is one of the biggest challenges in Baddha Konasana. But without the straight back, we do not experience the maximum benefit of the pose. These tricks can be done by those who sit on the floor and by those who sit on folded blankets.

All of my students have loved this trick. It is simple but with surprisingly pleasing results. After experiencing this trick, you will wish your Baddha Konasana could always be this good.

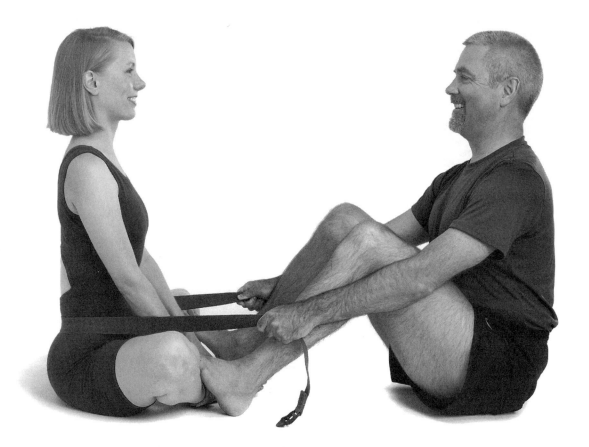

- Assume Baddha Konasana in the middle of the room.

- Have a friend sit in front of you with a strap (the thicker the better, but if all you have is a thin yoga strap or a necktie, that's fine).

- Your friend places the strap around your lower back, on the sacrum, and his feet on your shins.

- Your friend firmly and evenly pulls the strap toward him.

- See how much your back lifts and your knees go down? Doesn't it feel great? Be sure to return the favor.

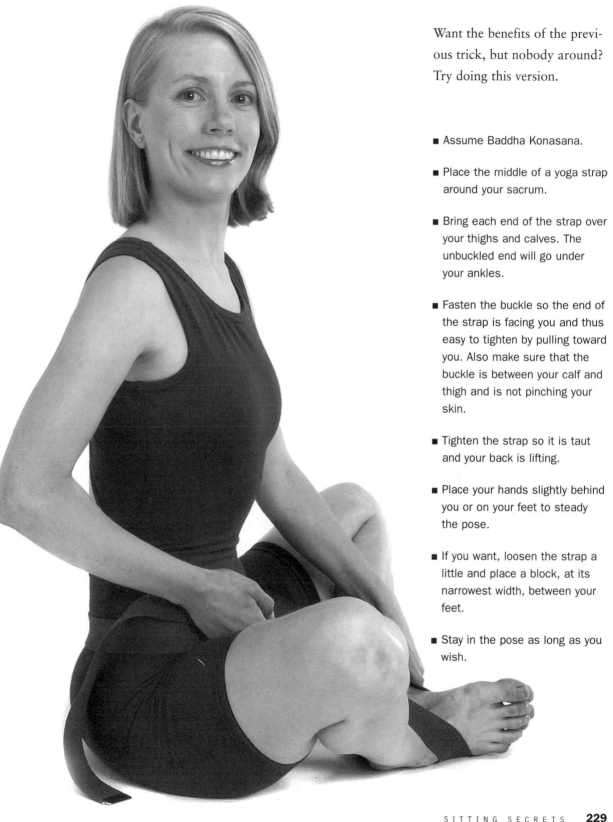

Want the benefits of the previous trick, but nobody around? Try doing this version.

- Assume Baddha Konasana.

- Place the middle of a yoga strap around your sacrum.

- Bring each end of the strap over your thighs and calves. The unbuckled end will go under your ankles.

- Fasten the buckle so the end of the strap is facing you and thus easy to tighten by pulling toward you. Also make sure that the buckle is between your calf and thigh and is not pinching your skin.

- Tighten the strap so it is taut and your back is lifting.

- Place your hands slightly behind you or on your feet to steady the pose.

- If you want, loosen the strap a little and place a block, at its narrowest width, between your feet.

- Stay in the pose as long as you wish.

PADMASANA

Lotus

Sitting in Padmasana increases circulation in the legs, lower abdomen, and lower back. Padmasana naturally lifts the spine and allows the body and mind to be simultaneously relaxed and alert. It is the traditional meditation posture.

- Sit with your legs extended in front of you.

- Bend your right leg and take hold of your knee and foot.

- Place your right foot on the top of your left thigh near the hip crease.

- Bend your left leg, hold your knee and foot, and place it on top of your right thigh near the hip crease.

- Bring your hands into prayer position or place the backs of your hands on your thighs.

- Hold the posture as long as you like. Release and switch leg positions. Place your left foot on the right thigh first, then place the right foot on the left thigh. The right leg will now be on top of the left leg.

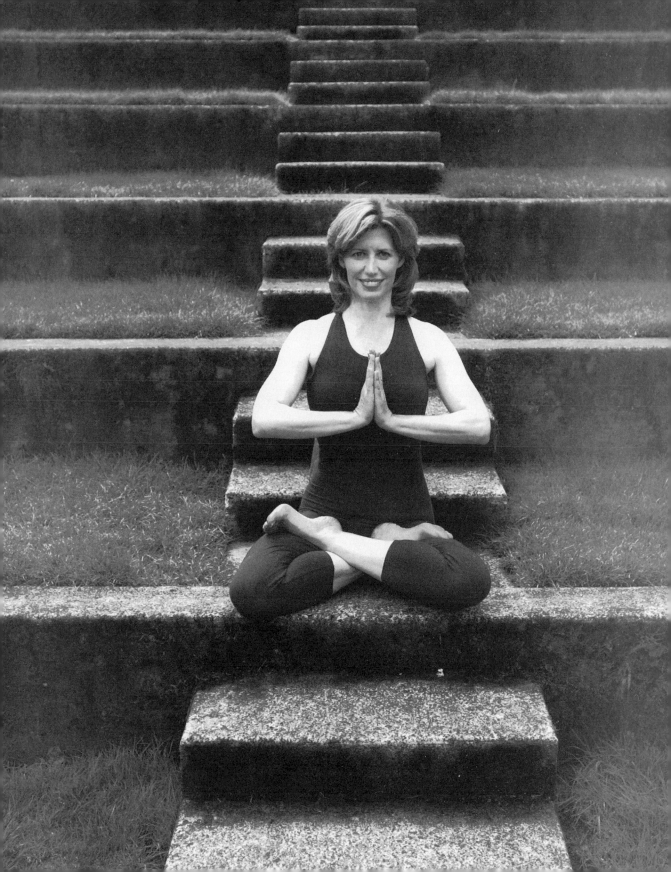

Named after the exquisite lotus flower, Padmasana makes most of us feel like sinking into the mud in which that flower grows. Most students cannot even approach the Lotus posture without excruciating pain in the knees and ankles. Sitting on a blanket and/or placing a strap or rolled face cloth behind the knees helps. Practicing Half Lotus is also a good way to ease into Full Lotus. But because the knee and ankle pain normally originates from tightness in the hips, it is best to approach Lotus carefully. Do not force yourself into this (or any pose) if you are not ready for it. A regular practice of standing poses and the other seated postures, along with the Lotus Prep Pose presented here, will ease your way to a more comfortable Padmasana.

Lotus Prep Pose

- Sit on the floor or on a folded blanket with your legs extended.

- Move your glutes aside so your sit bones are as close to the floor as possible.

- Bend your left leg and place your foot in front of you so it is aligned with the knee.

- Bend your right leg and place the side of that foot on top of your left knee.

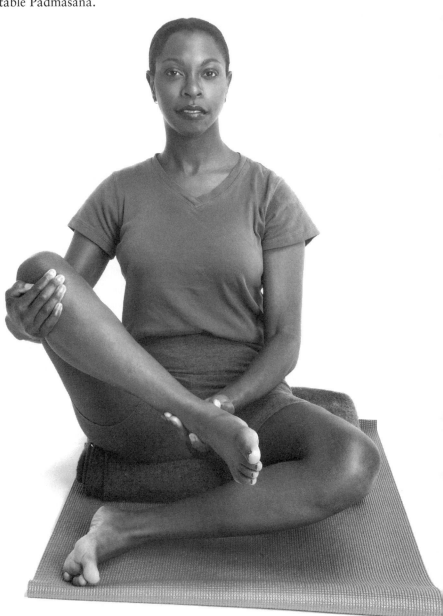

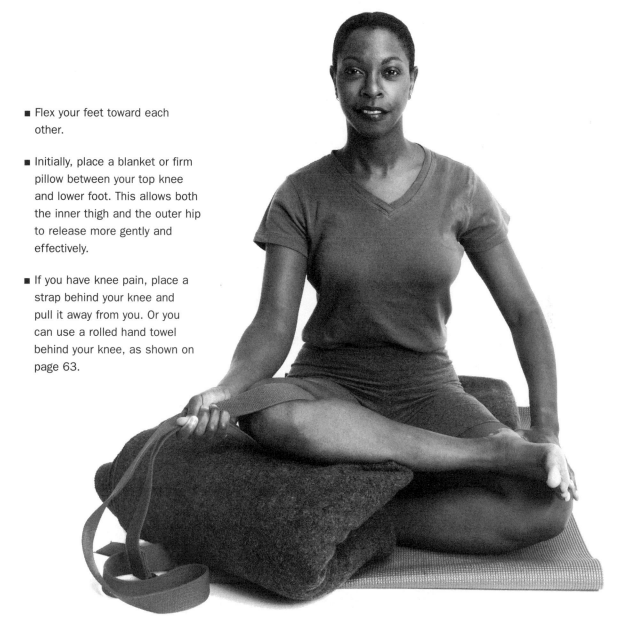

- Flex your feet toward each other.

- Initially, place a blanket or firm pillow between your top knee and lower foot. This allows both the inner thigh and the outer hip to release more gently and effectively.

- If you have knee pain, place a strap behind your knee and pull it away from you. Or you can use a rolled hand towel behind your knee, as shown on page 63.

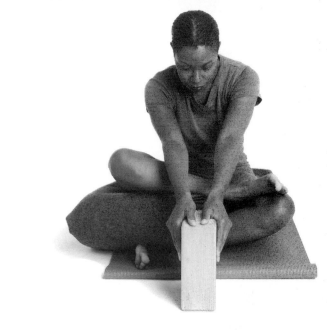

- To increase the stretch on the side of the hip, slowly move forward from your hip crease, placing your hands on a block.

- As the sides of your hips loosen, slowly move the block away from you. Eventually you will be able to put your forehead on the block.

- Carefully release and change your legs, placing the right leg on the floor and the left leg on top of it.

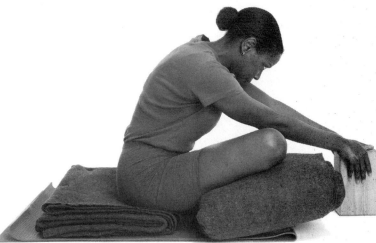

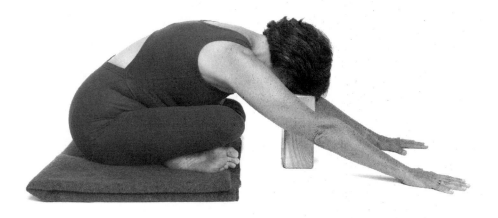

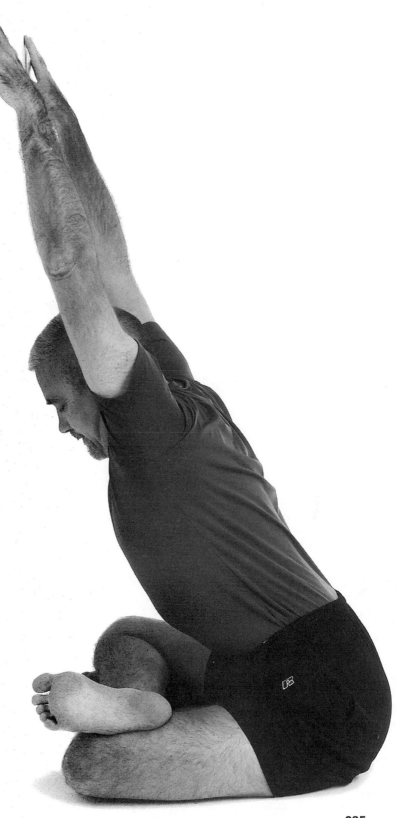

- In this version of Lotus Prep, assume the posture facing a wall. Make sure that the toes of each foot are touching the wall and are flexed toward each other.

- Walk your hands up the wall, lifting your arms as though you are lifting from the very lowest part of your back.

- Keeping the stretch intact, rest for a moment while your hips adjust. Then walk your hands higher. Continue the pattern of stretching, resting in the stretch, and extending the stretch several times.

- When you are finished, slowly release your legs and change the position of your legs.

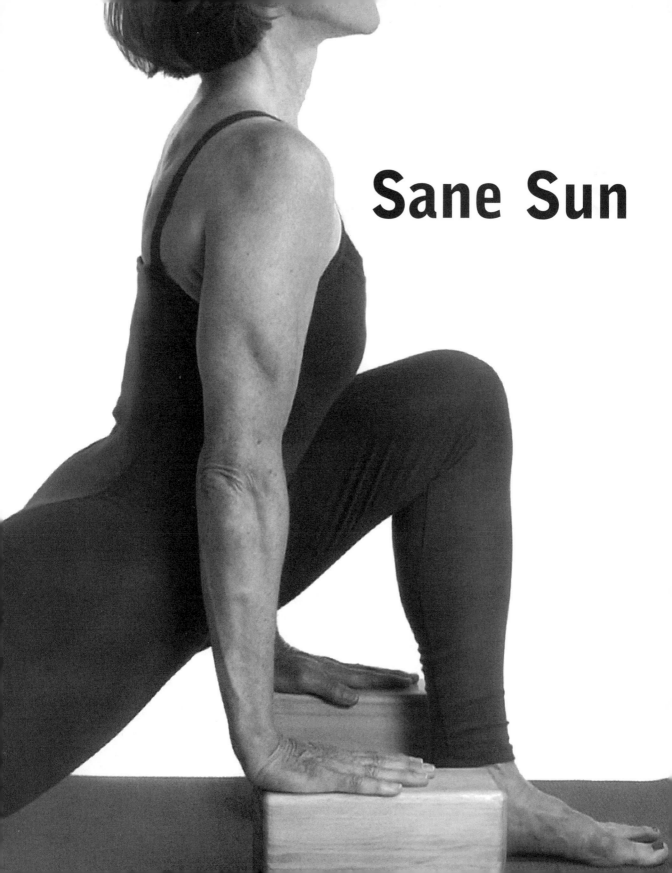

Sane Sun

Salutations

Sun Salutations are the basis of many yoga classes. They are invigorating and fun—but quite difficult for the beginning student. In this chapter, I offer some ways to practice Sun Salutations that help the beginner gain flexibility and strength and the ability to maintain appropriate musculoskeletal alignment. These Sun Salutations are much saner, safer, and more doable for beginners.

Different schools of yoga offer different ways to practice Sun Salutations. Alter this series to your own liking or to the way it is taught in the classes you attend.

Chair Sun Salutations

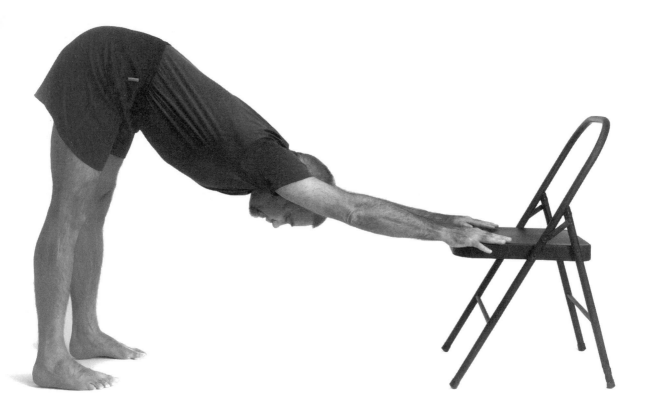

- To get started, place the back of a chair at the wall. If your shoulders are wide, use two chairs.

- Come into Downward-Facing Dog with your hands on the chair seat.

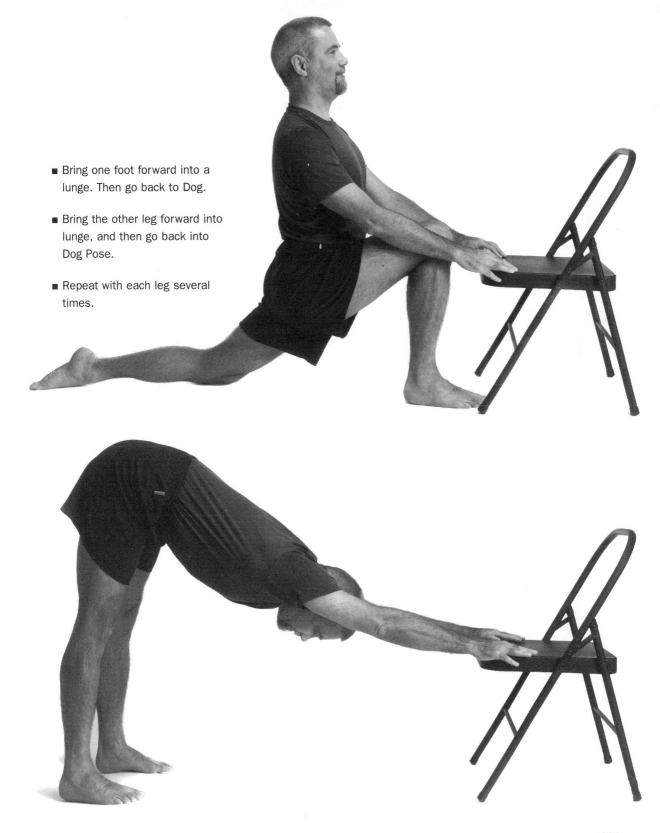

- Bring one foot forward into a lunge. Then go back to Dog.

- Bring the other leg forward into lunge, and then go back into Dog Pose.

- Repeat with each leg several times.

Phase II

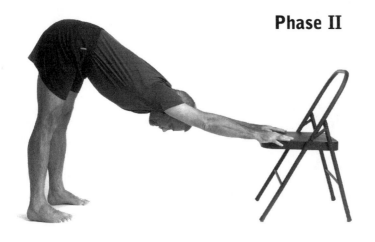

- Start in Chair Downward Dog.

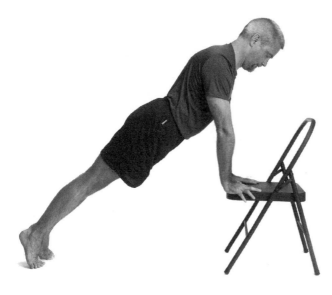

- Bring your shoulders over your hands so you are in Chair Plank Pose.

- Lift every arm muscle from your wrists to your shoulders.

- Firm your hips, lower back, lower abdomen, and legs. Hips stay in line with your spine.

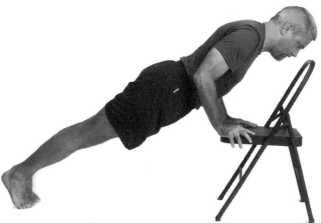

- Bend your elbows and lower your body into a modified push-up—Chair Chaturanga. Be cautious about your alignment. Hold for several seconds. If you like, you can repeat the Plank-Chaturanga combination several times. Or, if you prefer, you can skip Chaturanga.

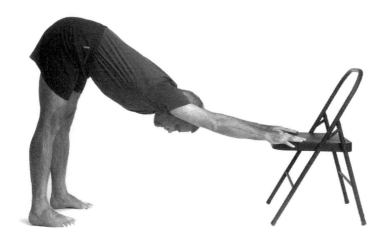

- Move back into Chair Downward Dog.

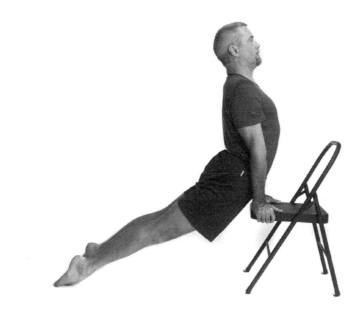

- Gently swing your body forward, bringing your pelvis to the edge of the chair seat.

- Puff your chest toward the wall as you arch your back.

- Your chest should be in front of your arms.

- Firm your hips, lower back, lower abdomen, and legs. Press the front and back of your body toward each other. Hold for several seconds.

- If you like, you can repeat the Downward Dog–Upward Dog combination several times.

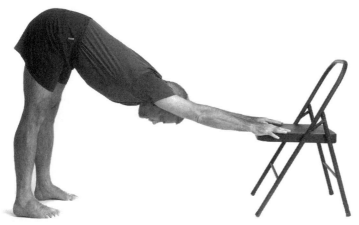

- Move back to Downward-Facing Dog

- Continue practicing the series as long as you like.

PUTTING IT ALL TOGETHER

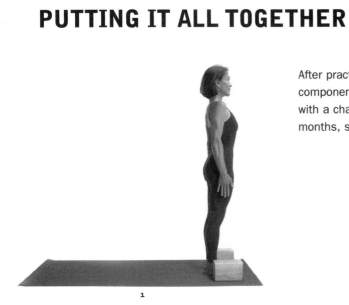

After practicing the various components of Sun Salutations with a chair for several weeks or months, switch to a pair of blocks.

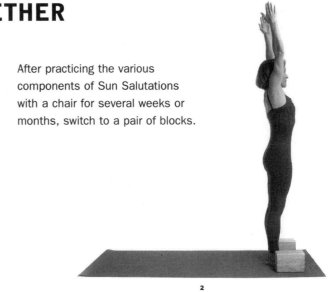

1

2

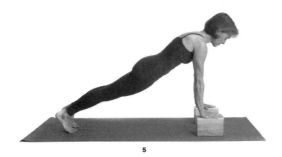

5

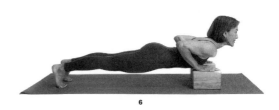

6

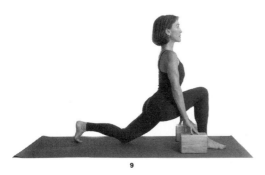

9

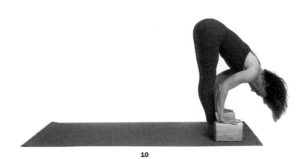

10

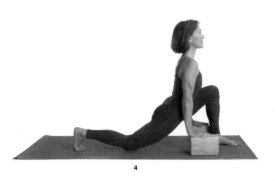

3

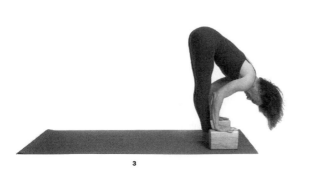

4

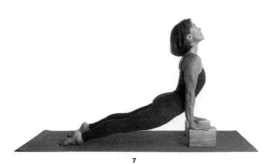

7

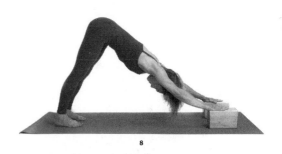

8

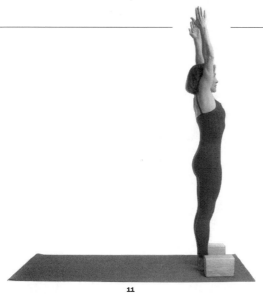

11

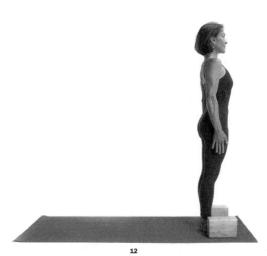

12

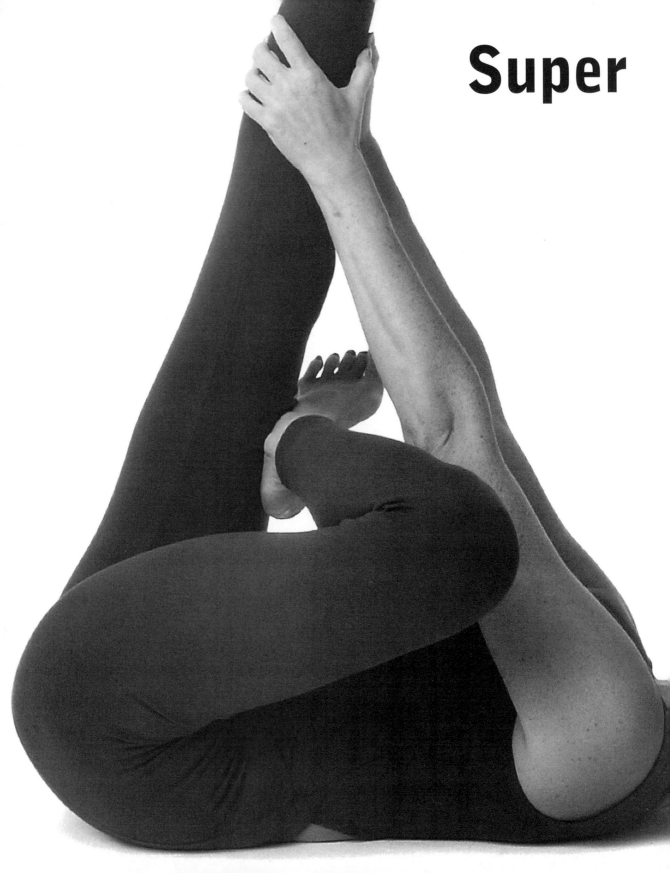

Super

Stretches

Sometimes we cannot perform the classic yoga postures because we simply do not have the required flexibility. For example, we cannot get the full benefit of a back bend if our shoulders are so tight that they don't allow for the complete extension of our arms. If our arms are not fully extended, our backs will not arch completely. Similarly, if our quadriceps and psoas muscles (the muscles that connect the spine and the thighbones) are tight, our backs will suffer. Furthermore, if our quads and psoas muscles are tight, we will look like a C in Headstand and Shoulder Stand rather than an I. And with tight hips, hamstrings, and quads, we certainly won't be able to do a split.

This chapter offers several "super stretches." This does not mean that you are expected to push yourself beyond your limits the very first time you try them. On the contrary, approach each stretch with gentleness and caution. It is much too easy to pull or tear a muscle if you move too deeply or too quickly into a stretch. You certainly don't want to elongate your muscles by pulling them. The goal is to gently coax your muscles to stretch a little bit more than normal. Each time you practice, move deeper into the stretch either by holding the pose longer or by more closely approximating the "ideal" stretch.

Every month or so, I teach a class that I call the "pre-split class." In it I teach some super stretches that help students go beyond their normal stretching limitations. In this class, students slowly stretch their muscles so that by the end of the class they can do a split—or at least come closer to doing a split than they could at the end of the previous pre-split class. Here are some of the stretches I teach in that class.

Knee-Up-the-Wall Pose

Caution: *You may want to practice some of your normal stretches prior to attempting these super stretches.*

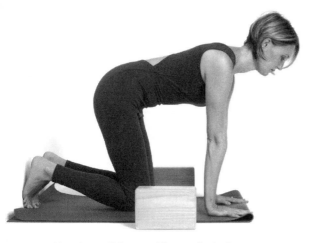

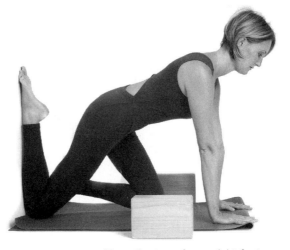

- Kneel on all fours with your feet at a wall. Have a chair or two yoga blocks near your side in case you need them for support.

- Place the top of your right foot on the wall and slide your knee so it is against the wall. Your shin is now on the wall.

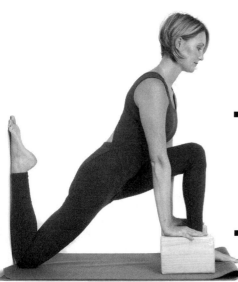

- Holding on to a chair or yoga blocks for support, if necessary, bring your left foot out and place the sole of the foot on the floor so your ankle and knee are aligned.

- Assess the feeling in your right hamstring. If you think you can stretch more, go deeper into the lunge. Hold the chair, some blocks, or place your hands on the floor if that feels safe.

- Do not push the stretch; allow gravity to gently lengthen your muscles.

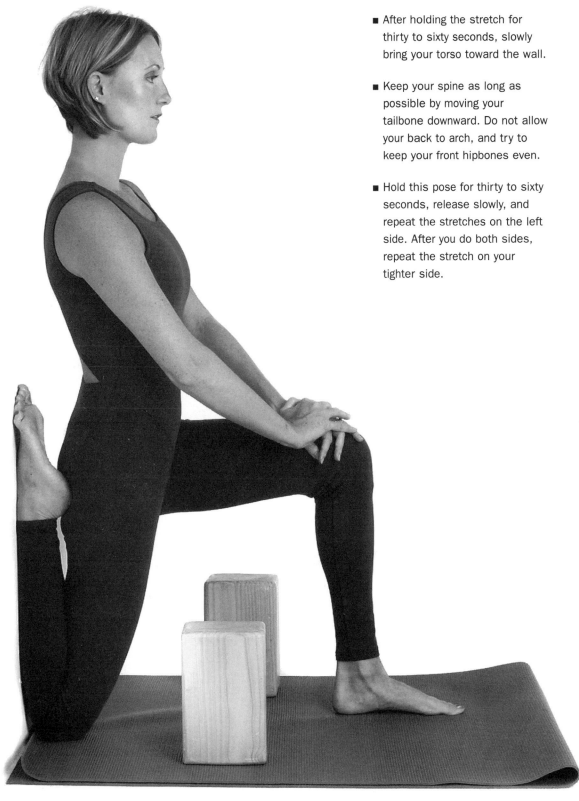

- After holding the stretch for thirty to sixty seconds, slowly bring your torso toward the wall.

- Keep your spine as long as possible by moving your tailbone downward. Do not allow your back to arch, and try to keep your front hipbones even.

- Hold this pose for thirty to sixty seconds, release slowly, and repeat the stretches on the left side. After you do both sides, repeat the stretch on your tighter side.

Half Supta Virasana

Caution: *If you normally sit on a block or blanket in Virasana, skip this stretch.*

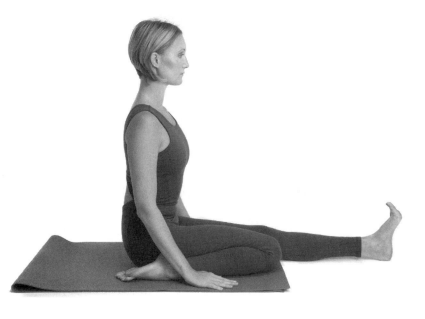

- Sit on the floor with your legs stretched out, feet together.

- You may want a prop behind you: a rolled yoga mat, folded blankets, or a bolster.

- With your hands, release your glutes outward so your sit bones are as close to the floor as possible.

- Bend your right leg so your shin is on the floor, your calf is next to your thigh, and your foot is next to your hip.

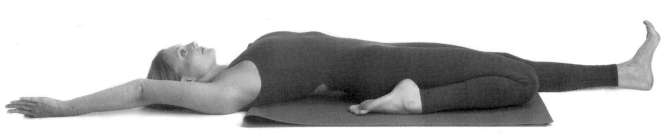

- Bend your extended knee and place the sole of your foot on the floor as you slowly lie down. You can then extend that leg again.

- Press your bent knee into the floor.

- Assess the stretch. If you want to augment it, bring your right hand overhead and stretch it away from you.

- To further intensify your stretch, bring your left knee into your chest and hold it with both your hands. Or, you can hold it with your left hand and bring your right hand overhead again.

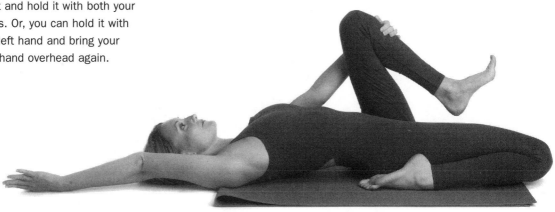

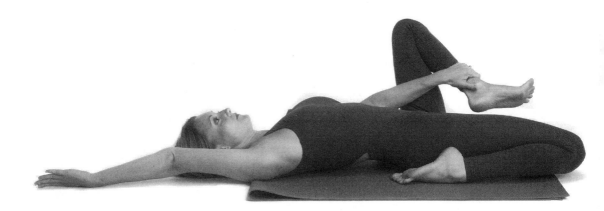

- To go beyond that intensity, clasp your left ankle with your left hand and lower your leg to the side. Hold as long as you wish before bringing your leg back to center.

- If you like, you can place a sandbag on your thigh that is in Virasana or have a friend hold your leg, as shown in the Supta Virasana series.

- Hold each phase of the pose as long as you like.

- Release your pose, and repeat the series with your left leg in Virasana.

Supta Virasana

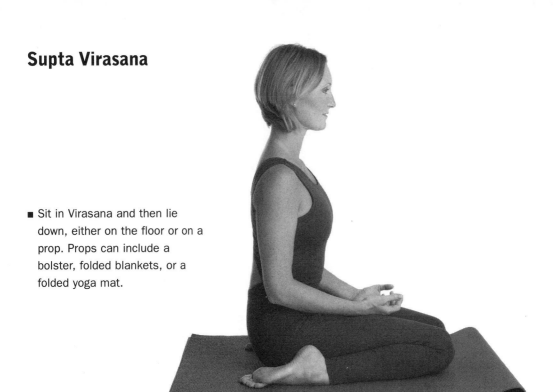

- Sit in Virasana and then lie down, either on the floor or on a prop. Props can include a bolster, folded blankets, or a folded yoga mat.

- To intensify the stretch, have a friend firmly press your thighs downward.

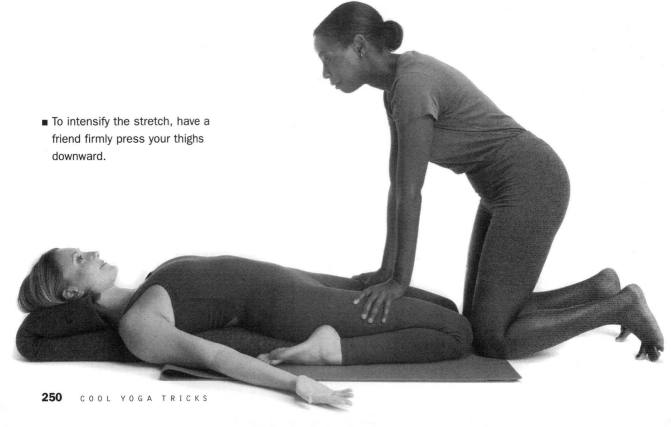

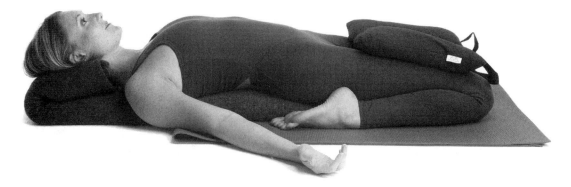

■ Or, place a sandbag on each thigh.

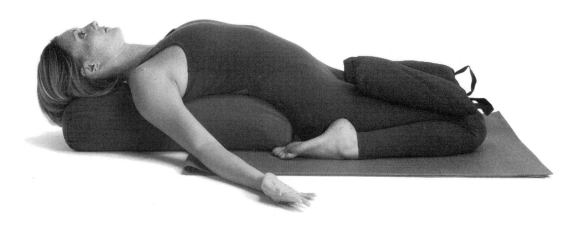

■ Relax and lengthen your lower back and hip muscles and extend them toward your knees (think of moving your tailbone toward your knees and try to actualize that movement).

■ Rest in this pose as long as you like.

INTENSE HAMSTRING STRETCHES

Block Stretch

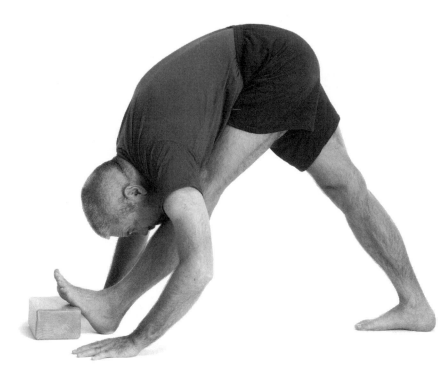

- Center a block near the end of your yoga mat, laying it flat.

- Stand about two feet from the block. Bring your left foot around and place the ball of your foot on the block. Engage both sets of quadriceps.

- From the hip crease, slowly lean forward. Align your front hipbones so they are even.

- Progressively move your abdomen down your leg, allowing your hamstring to slowly release. Place your hands on the floor if you can.

- To intensify the stretch:

  - flex the toes of your forward foot toward you

  - lift your back heel

- If the stretch is too intense:

  - place a yoga block on each side of your forward foot and hold them with your hands

- Slowly come out of the pose and switch sides.

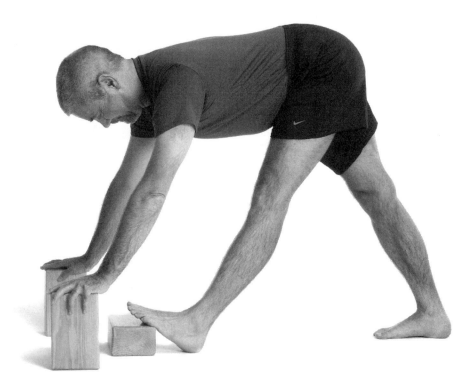

Uttanasana with Your Back at the Wall

- Stand facing a wall, a few inches away.

- With your feet a little wider than hip-distance apart, bend forward into Uttanasana.

- Walk toward the wall and place your back against the wall.

- Stay in this pose for thirty to sixty seconds. Then slide your back down the wall.

- Hold for thirty to sixty seconds and then slide your back down the wall again.

- Continue in this mode for several minutes.

- Release, rest for a moment, and try again.

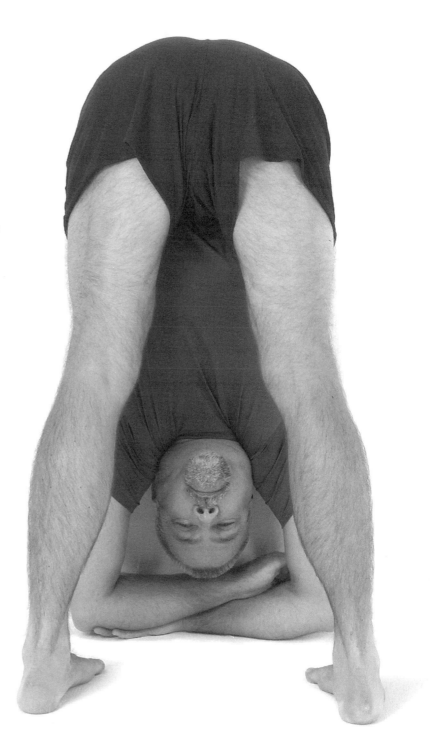

Wall Split

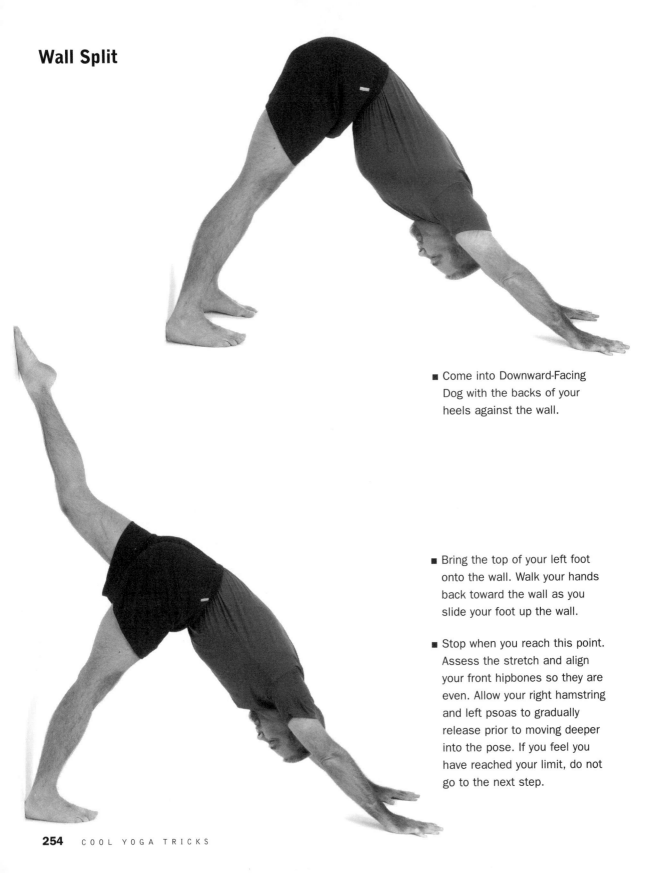

- Come into Downward-Facing Dog with the backs of your heels against the wall.

- Bring the top of your left foot onto the wall. Walk your hands back toward the wall as you slide your foot up the wall.

- Stop when you reach this point. Assess the stretch and align your front hipbones so they are even. Allow your right hamstring and left psoas to gradually release prior to moving deeper into the pose. If you feel you have reached your limit, do not go to the next step.

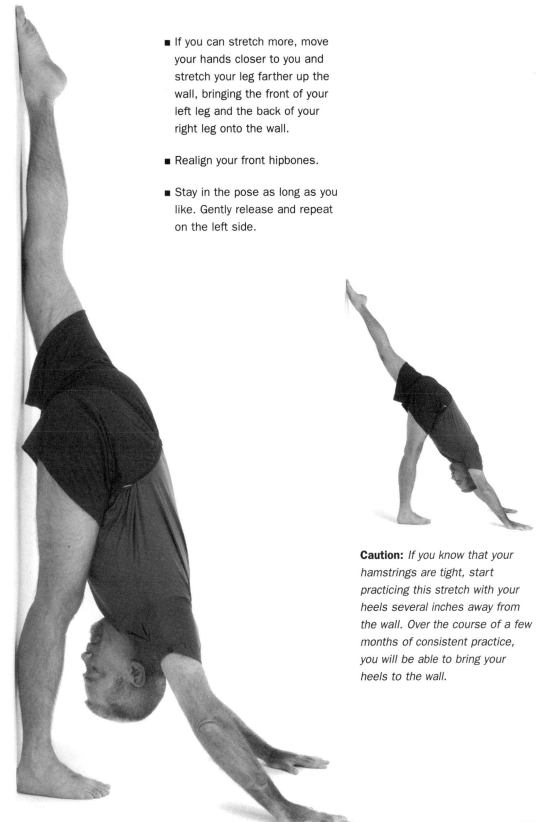

- If you can stretch more, move your hands closer to you and stretch your leg farther up the wall, bringing the front of your left leg and the back of your right leg onto the wall.

- Realign your front hipbones.

- Stay in the pose as long as you like. Gently release and repeat on the left side.

Caution: *If you know that your hamstrings are tight, start practicing this stretch with your heels several inches away from the wall. Over the course of a few months of consistent practice, you will be able to bring your heels to the wall.*

HIP STRETCHES

- Lie down and bring your right leg into Lotus, or as close to Lotus as you can.

- Straighten your left leg and slowly pull it toward you. Allow the muscles to release gradually. Breathe into the tight muscles. As you are ready, gradually pull your leg closer to you.

- Release and switch sides.

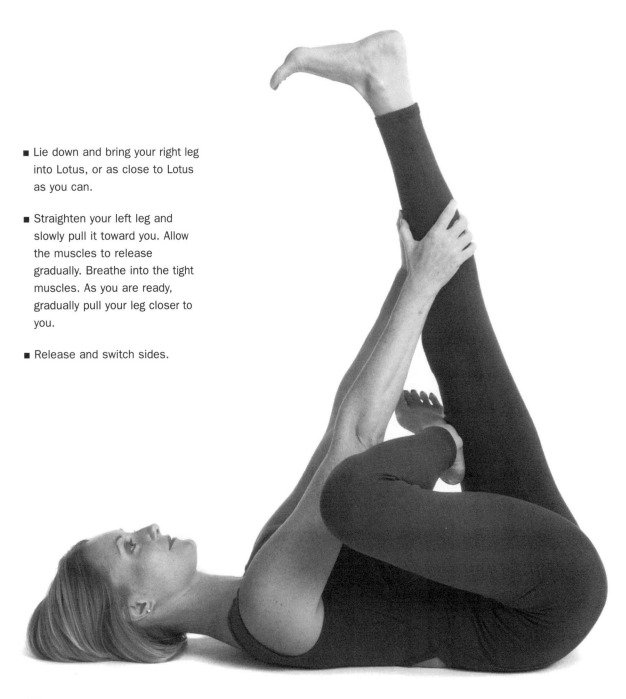

■ Repeat each side with the
non-Lotus leg bent instead
of straight.

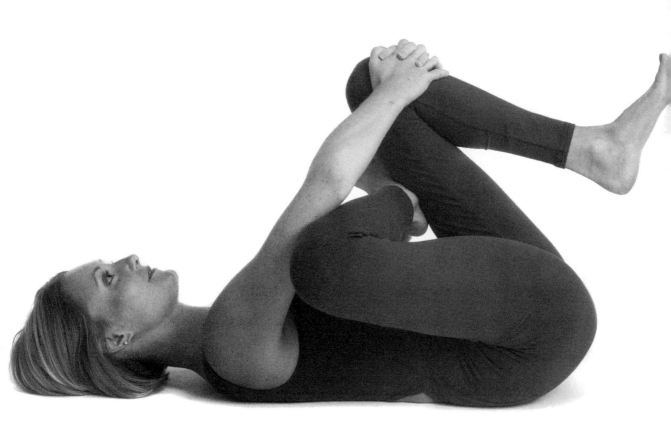

Pre–King Pigeon Pose

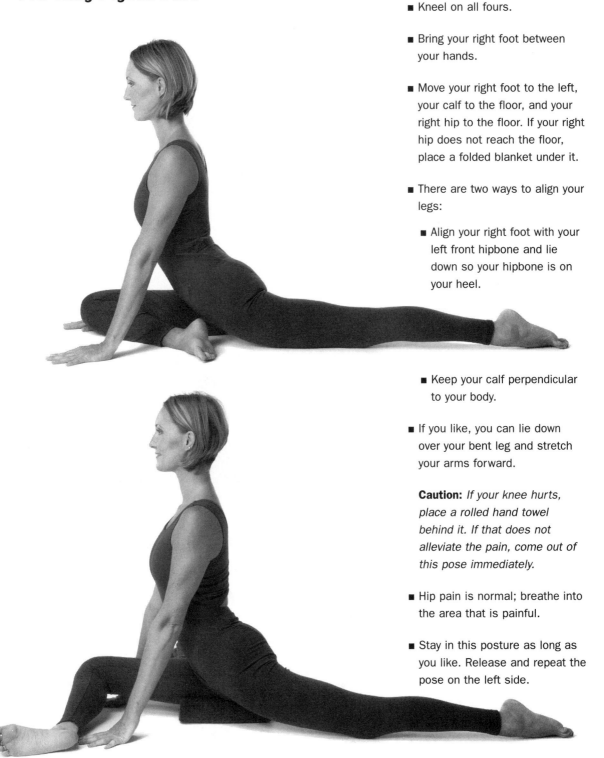

- Kneel on all fours.

- Bring your right foot between your hands.

- Move your right foot to the left, your calf to the floor, and your right hip to the floor. If your right hip does not reach the floor, place a folded blanket under it.

- There are two ways to align your legs:

  - Align your right foot with your left front hipbone and lie down so your hipbone is on your heel.

- Keep your calf perpendicular to your body.

- If you like, you can lie down over your bent leg and stretch your arms forward.

Caution: *If your knee hurts, place a rolled hand towel behind it. If that does not alleviate the pain, come out of this pose immediately.*

- Hip pain is normal; breathe into the area that is painful.

- Stay in this posture as long as you like. Release and repeat the pose on the left side.

Block Split

When you are ready to try a split, but not sure you have the flexibility yet, try this trick.

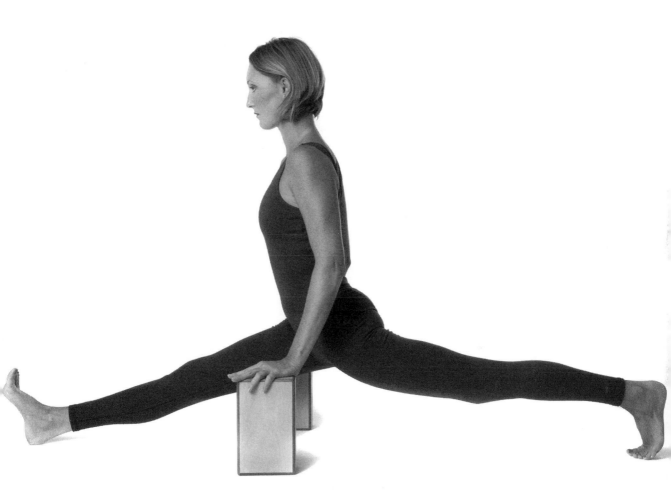

- Kneel on all fours with blocks under your hands.

- Step your right foot forward and slide it as far forward as you can. Stretch your left leg back.

- Bring your left hipbone forward and your right hipbone backward so they are aligned.

- Continue to straighten both legs and lower your hips.

- Go as far as you can for this session, release, and repeat the pose with your left leg forward.

SUPER SHOULDER STRETCHES

Super Shoulder Stretches are necessary to gain the required flexibility for many inversions and back bends. Slowly and cautiously, try these tricks for newfound shoulder suppleness.

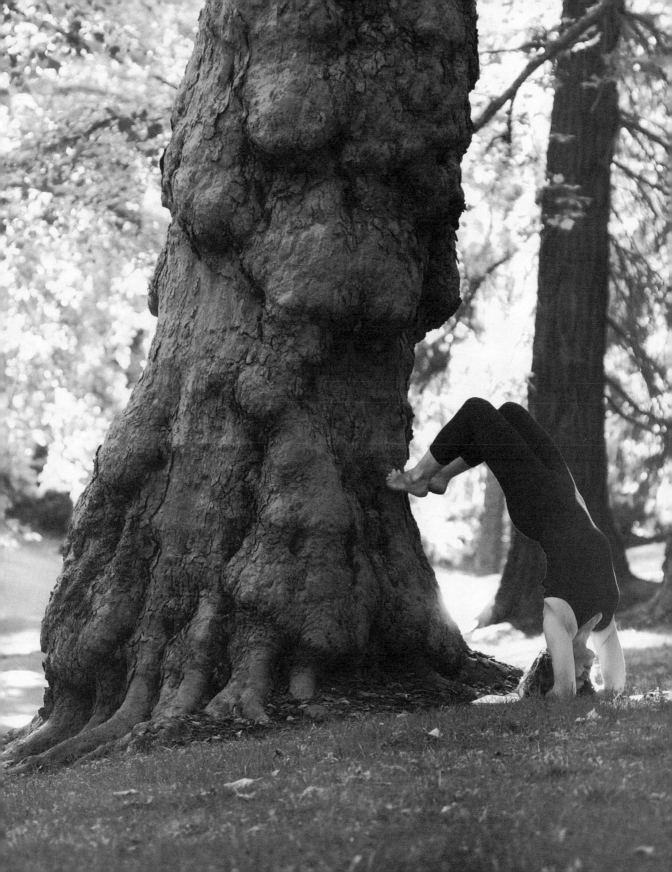

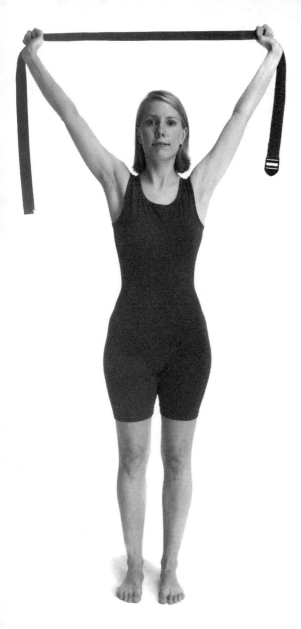
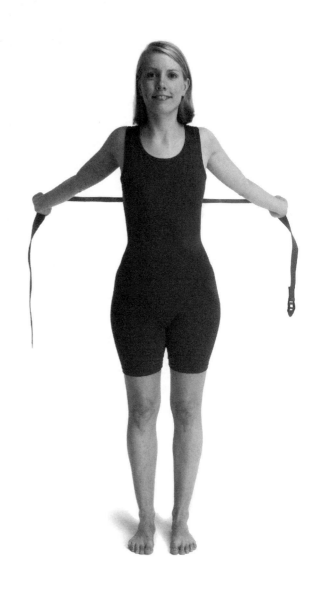

Shoulder Rotation

- With your hands placed several inches wider than your shoulders, hold a yoga strap, exercise band, necktie, bathrobe belt, or broom handle above your head.

- Rotate the outside edges of your armpits and your deltoid muscles forward.

- Bring your hands behind you, widening them if necessary. If you are using an exercise band, there will be no need to widen your hands. If you are using a yoga strap, be sure to keep it taut.

- If your shoulders are very tight, initially you may not be able to bring the strap all the way back. This will improve as you practice the stretch.

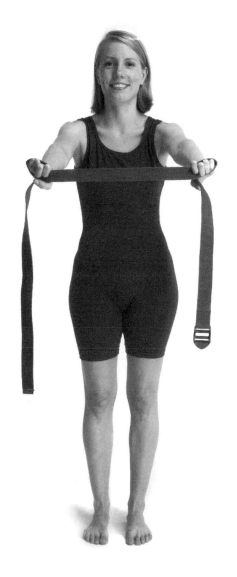

- Move the strap back to center. Roll the outside edges of your armpits and deltoid muscles forward.

- Then bring your arms in front of you (narrow your hands on the strap if necessary). Exaggerate the move so your shoulders and upper back are rounded. Then move your arms so the strap is centered overhead again. Rotate the outside edges of your armpits and deltoid muscles forward and bring the arms behind you again.

- Continue in this mode as long as you like, making sure that each time you reach center you roll the outside edges of your armpits and deltoid muscles forward.

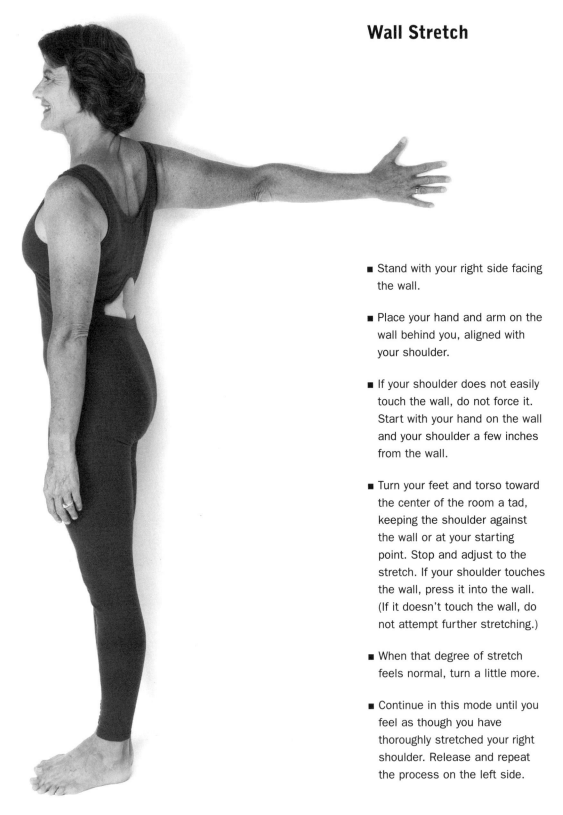

Wall Stretch

- Stand with your right side facing the wall.

- Place your hand and arm on the wall behind you, aligned with your shoulder.

- If your shoulder does not easily touch the wall, do not force it. Start with your hand on the wall and your shoulder a few inches from the wall.

- Turn your feet and torso toward the center of the room a tad, keeping the shoulder against the wall or at your starting point. Stop and adjust to the stretch. If your shoulder touches the wall, press it into the wall. (If it doesn't touch the wall, do not attempt further stretching.)

- When that degree of stretch feels normal, turn a little more.

- Continue in this mode until you feel as though you have thoroughly stretched your right shoulder. Release and repeat the process on the left side.

Shoulder Blade Stretches

The primary purpose of these stretches is to expand the back shoulder muscles. But do not be surprised if you find that all of your shoulder muscles get stretched.

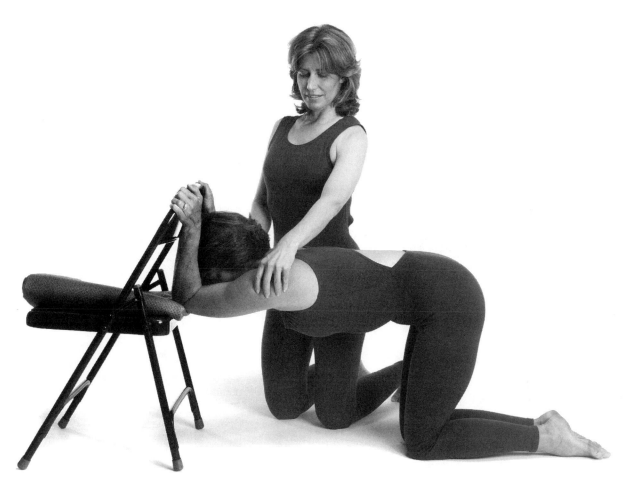

- Place a folded yoga mat on a chair seat.

- Kneel behind the chair. Place your elbows, as close together as possible, on the chair seat and your hands on the top of the chairback.

- Walk your knees back so your torso is parallel to the floor and

your thighs and torso are at a right angle to each other.

- Keep the front of your torso moving in toward your back so that your back does not collapse downward.

- Press your elbows into the chair and roll the outside edge of

your armpits and deltoid muscles toward the floor.

- You can also have a friend roll your deltoids for you so your body can learn, and remember, the movement.

- Hold as long as you like. Rest for a moment and try the next two stretches.

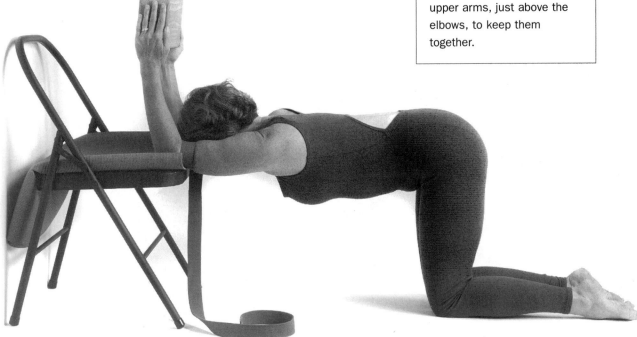

Note for all three stretches:

When you have increased your flexibility to the point that you can do this pose with your elbows next to each other, tie a strap around your upper arms, just above the elbows, to keep them together.

- Kneel in front of the chair, holding a block between your hands.

- Place your elbows on the chair seat, as close together as possible. Place a strap above your elbows, if you like, close enough together to create some challenge. (See Note.)

- Walk your knees back so your torso is parallel to the floor and your thighs and torso are at a right angle to each other.

- Keep the front of your torso moving in toward your back so that your back does not collapse downward.

- Press your elbows into the chair and roll the outside edge of your armpits and deltoid muscles toward the floor.

- Hold as long as you like. Rest for a moment and try the next stretch.

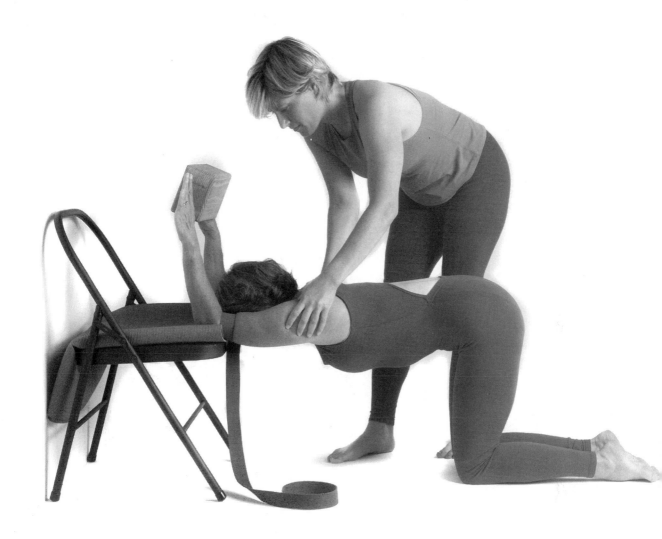

- In this version, have a friend place a block between your thumbs and forefingers.

- Your friend then rolls the outside edge of your armpits and your deltoid muscles toward the floor.

- Be sure to keep your neck relaxed throughout the stretch, resting your face on your upper arms or on the strap if you like.

- Hold this stretch as long as you like and have your friend help you release from the pose.

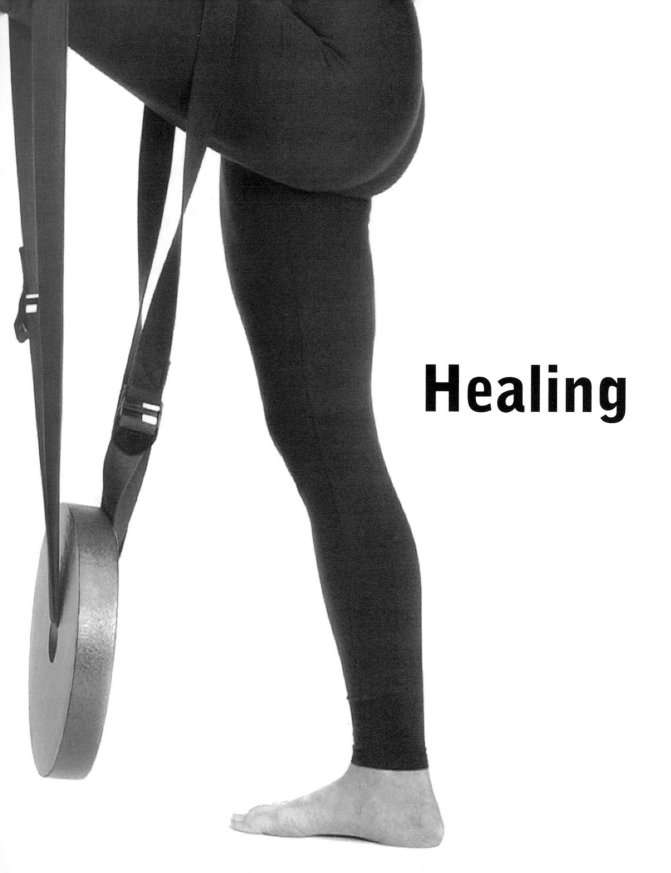

Healing

the Hurts

We all know that yoga both prevents and heals myriad physical problems. While my knowledge is limited, it is evident that yoga promotes healing by stimulating the body's immune system and its own healing mechanisms. B.K.S. Iyengar has been at the forefront of yoga therapy for more than fifty years. My knowledge on this subject comes from his tradition. My presentation here is in no way a comprehensive treatise on yoga therapy. In fact, it is much more of a hodgepodge of tricks that I have used for myself and for my students—all with great results.

Through a regular practice of yoga, some of my students with asthma, fibromyalgia, and lupus have dispensed with their medication completely. Many students with serious arthritis, herniated discs, and neck and back injuries have enjoyed tremendous pain relief through yoga. After the publication of my first book, *Yoga for Wimps,* several women with partial leg amputations e-mailed me with the news that they were able to do yoga from my book. One woman wrote that her entire amputee support group was practicing yoga from the book. People with cancer wrote, telling me that practicing yoga made them feel better emotionally and gave them more stamina. Men who had been forced to give up their favorite sports due to pain were grateful that once again they were able to enjoy running, biking, and golfing. Many of the e-mails I received brought tears to my eyes.

I am very grateful to Mr. Iyengar and that his knowledge, disseminated through me, has helped so many people. Mr. Iyengar and his students throughout the world are helping to heal people each and every day. If you are interested in learning more about yoga and healing, please refer to Mr. Iyengar's books: *Light on Yoga* and *Yoga: The Path to Holistic Health.*

If you have some simple ailments, this chapter may help you experience relief. If you have more serious problems, please consult with your physician.

Forehead to Block Pose

There are few techniques that stop pounding headaches and relieve neck and shoulder pain as quickly as this one does. It also quiets a chattering mind. This is a restorative pose and if you are not 100 percent comfortable, try another posture. If you don't have the flexibility to use a block, place your forehead on a chair seat.

- Sit in a comfortable position (wide angle, straight-legged, or cross-legged) in front of a yoga block.

- Close your eyes and place your forehead—the area between your eyebrows—on the block.

- Keep your hands in front of the block and allow your shoulders to relax.

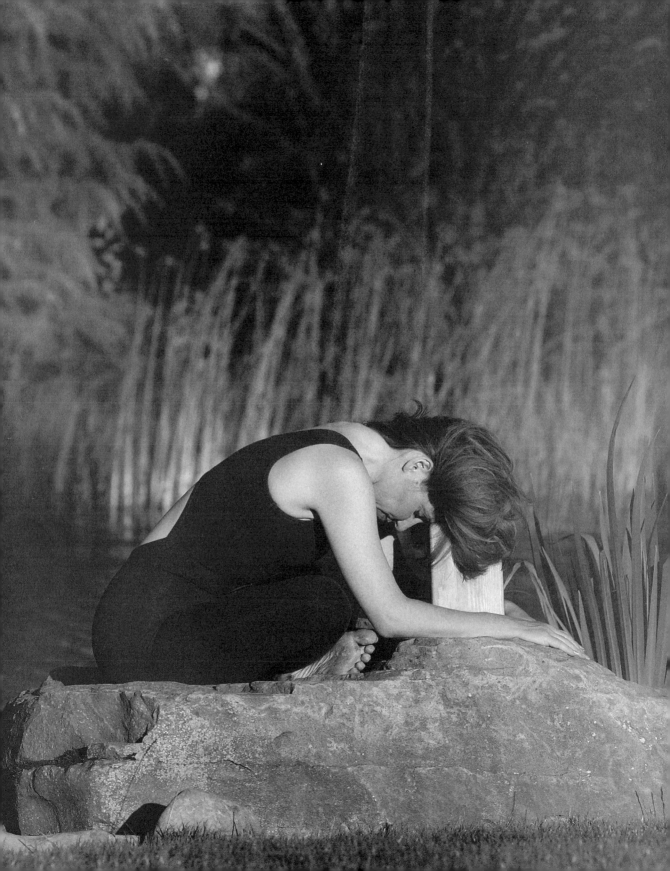

HEADACHES AND NECKACHES

Headaches and neckaches are easy to resolve through yoga. I know this all too well. Here are some additional ways that you can heal your headache, whether it is a regular tension headache, a migraine, or a result of sinus problems.

Head Support Pose

This pose allows your mind to quiet quickly and also helps relieve headaches and neckaches.

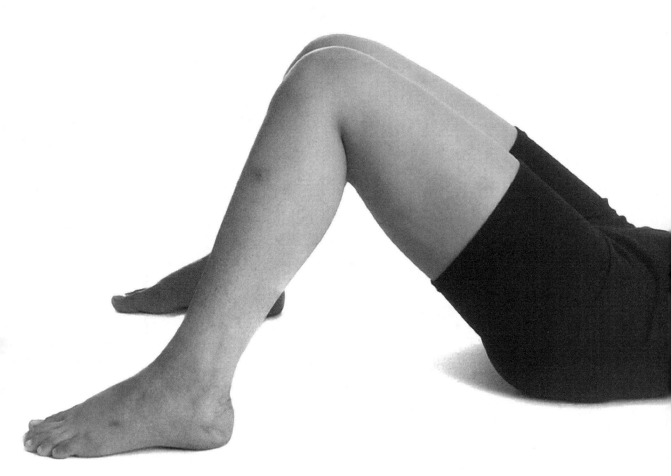

- Lie down and place the back of your head on a yoga block.

- Bend your knees, allowing them to touch each other. Your feet should be a little wider than your hips.

- If you don't feel completely relaxed, try a thicker or thinner prop (such as a book).

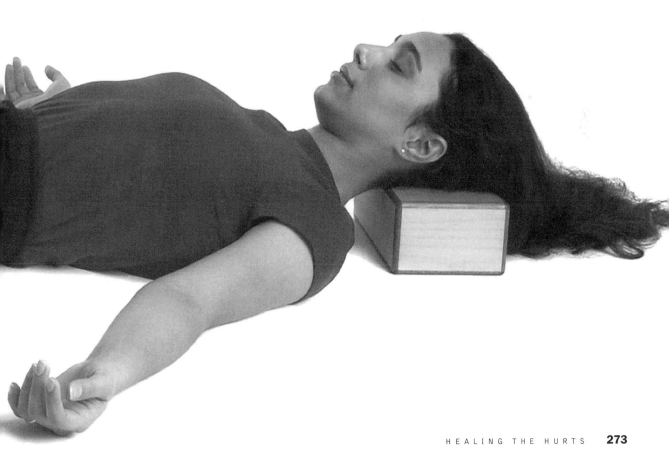

The Ace Bandage Technique

Wrapping an Ace bandage around your head may cause your friends and family to question your sanity. But if you have a headache that won't go away, try this, and by the time the men in the white coats arrive at your door, your headache will be gone.

One of my students used to suffer regularly from migraines. In late 2001, I taught him this technique. He uses it as soon as he feels a headache coming on. The relief is immediate, he says, and he has not had a migraine since.

Wrap your head with the Ace bandage and then assume one of your favorite restorative postures.

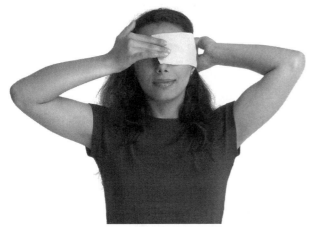

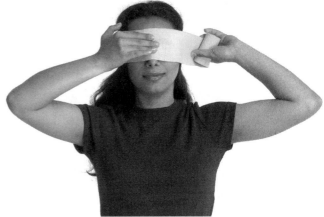

- Start with the Ace bandage rolled and your eyes closed.

- Take the end and place it between your eyebrows, covering part of the bridge of your nose and part of your forehead.

- Holding the end with one hand, partially unroll the bandage and cover one eye.

- Wrap the bandage around the back of your head and then cover the second eye and then the first eye again.

- The bandage wrap is even at this point and you no longer need to hold the end.

- As you bring the bandage around the back of your head again, angle the roll upward on the back of your head and then use a downward stroke to cover both eyes.

- On the third layer, angle the bandage downward on the back of your head and sweep the layer upward as you cover your eyes.

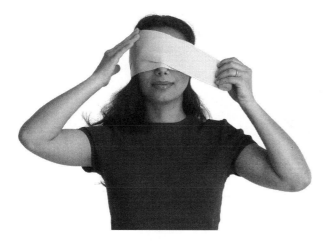

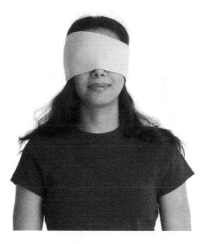

- Continue bandaging your head in this manner until you finish the roll.

- When you come to the end of the roll, tuck it into the bandage on the side of your head.

- Keep your eyes closed and allow the eyelids to be soft.

- Place your index fingers under the bandage, starting at the top of your nose, then slide your fingers across your eyelids. This evens out the skin underneath the bandage.

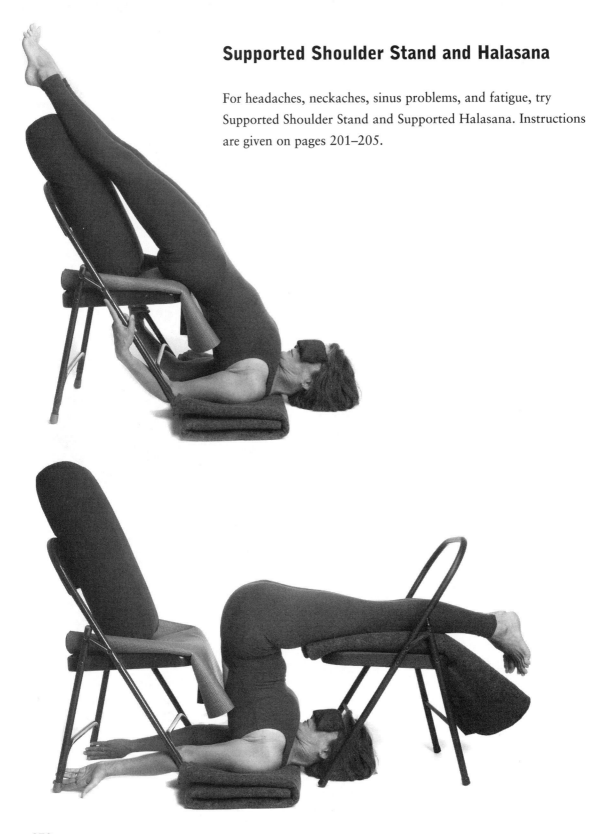

Supported Shoulder Stand and Halasana

For headaches, neckaches, sinus problems, and fatigue, try
Supported Shoulder Stand and Supported Halasana. Instructions
are given on pages 201–205.

Supported Uttanasana

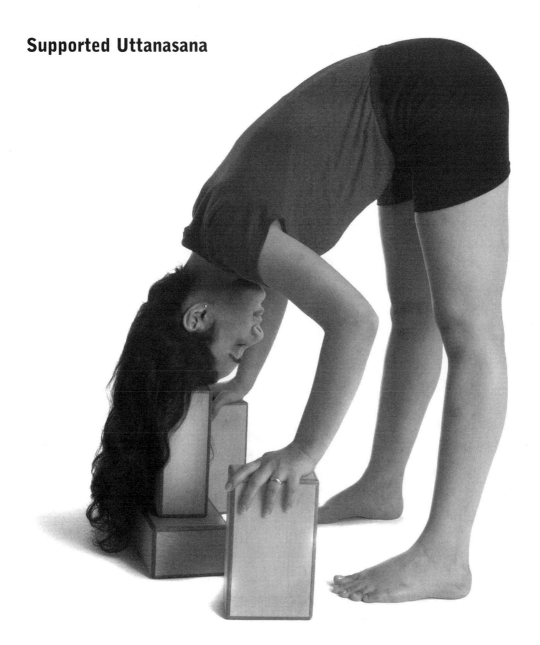

- Stack two to four blocks as shown.

- Place a block on each side of the stack.

- Stand about a foot from the stack with your legs separated by about eighteen inches.

- Lean forward from your hip crease and place the crown of your head on the stack.

- Hold each side block with your hands or place your forearms on the blocks.

- Hold as long as you like, relaxing into the pose.

RELIEF FOR COLDS, FLU, FATIGUE, HIGH BLOOD PRESSURE, TUMMYACHES, AND MENSTRUAL CRAMPS

Restorative back bends relieve myriad problems. See pages 131 to 133 for alternative restorative postures.

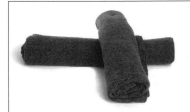

Arrange your blankets this way. Place as many or as few blankets as you need under your head to be completely comfortable.

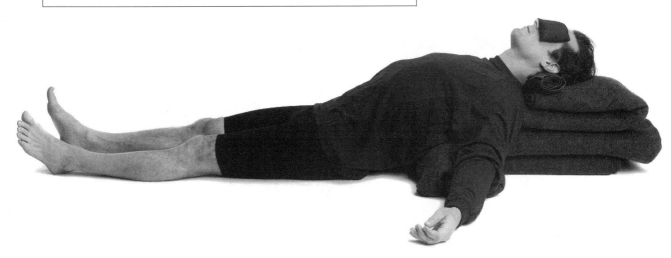

- Fold two blankets into quarters and roll them. Place one blanket lengthwise and the other across it. Or you can use two bolsters and place one crosswise over the other.

- Sit in front of the blanket setup, with your lower back directly against the props, and lie down. Adjust the crosswise blanket or bolster so it is directly behind your sternum.

- Use a blanket to support your head or a rolled hand towel to support your neck.

- Make sure you are 100 percent comfortable. If not, adjust the thickness of your props.

- Stay in the pose as long as you like (I usually fall asleep), using an eye cover and earplugs to block out the light and noise.

- See blanket bends on pages 131–133 for more restorative back bends.

KNEE PROBLEMS

Knee problems come in many different forms and are caused by different things. However, one thing that most knee problems have in common is that the real problem is in the hips, ankles, or feet, and the knee takes the brunt of it.

I got very serious about my yoga practice after a knee injury that resulted in surgery. The surgery and the physical therapy did not take away the pain. The committed yoga practice did. Here are a few of the tricks that helped that process. But remember: Knees are delicate and you should always consult your physician before you attempt yoga therapy.

Strengthening the Muscles Around the Knee

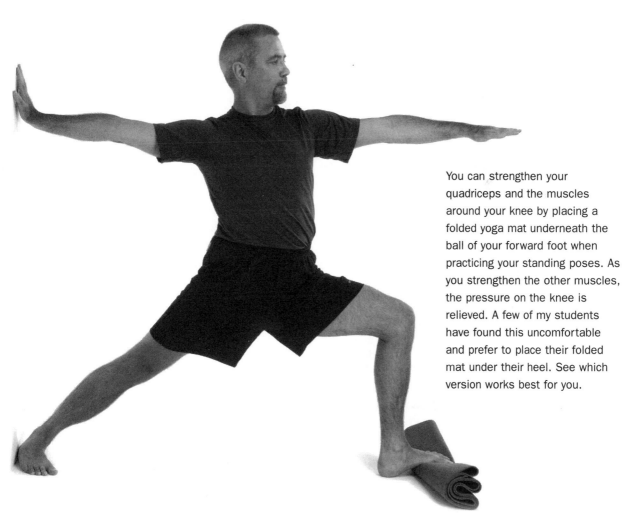

You can strengthen your quadriceps and the muscles around your knee by placing a folded yoga mat underneath the ball of your forward foot when practicing your standing poses. As you strengthen the other muscles, the pressure on the knee is relieved. A few of my students have found this uncomfortable and prefer to place their folded mat under their heel. See which version works best for you.

Virasana Tricks

When I committed to yoga to help heal my knee pain, several teachers mentioned that the only yoga posture that Mr. Iyengar guarantees is Virasana. Apparently, the guarantee is that if you practice this pose for ten minutes or more each day, it will heal your knee problems. Sitting in this pose increases flexibility in your hips, ankles, and feet. But, of course, if your knees are stiff you will need to sit on a lift.

Virasana is also a godsend for circulation problems, varicose veins, and heel spurs.

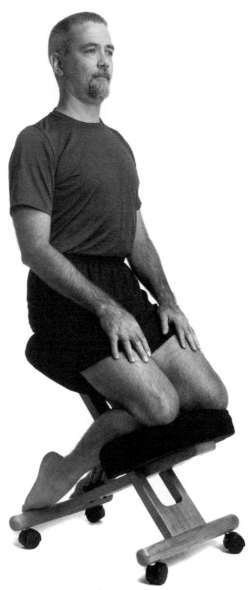

I have had many students who are so stiff that they cannot sit on a block or a couple of thick phone books to get started. Thus, I have them sit in a kneeling chair for Virasana. One student healed her painful heel spurs within a few weeks of diligent Virasana practice in the kneeling chair.

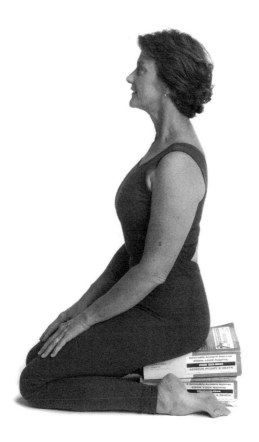 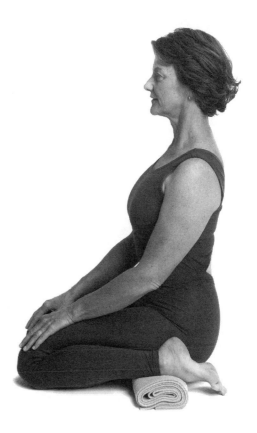

If you are stiff, but still flexible enough to sit close to the floor, sit on very thick phone books. During my knee-therapy phase I was living in Denver, and I started out on two Denver telephone books. As I gained flexibility, I would tear a few pages out of a book. Within about eight months, I was able to sit on the floor.

When I moved to a rural environment, I had to change my prescription to using two very thick books that I didn't mind tearing up. You can also use a yoga block, a yoga block with a thinner book under it, or a yoga block with a folded blanket on top.

To increase flexibility in your feet and ankles, try placing a folded mat under your metatarsals. After sitting with the mat or blanket under your metatarsals, move the prop closer to your toes. This variation is great for runners and for people who get cramps in their feet and ankles.

LOWER BACK PAIN

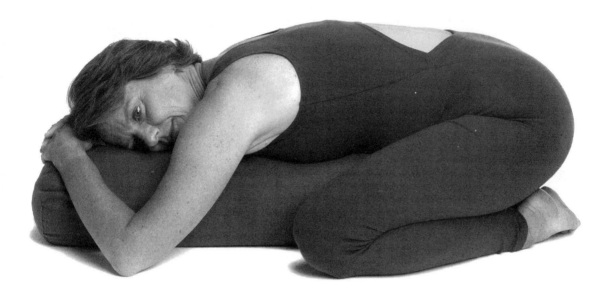

Supported Child's Pose

■ Kneel with your legs wide apart.
Place some folded blankets,
bolsters, or firm pillows
between your legs.

■ Come into Child's Pose and rest
as long as you like.

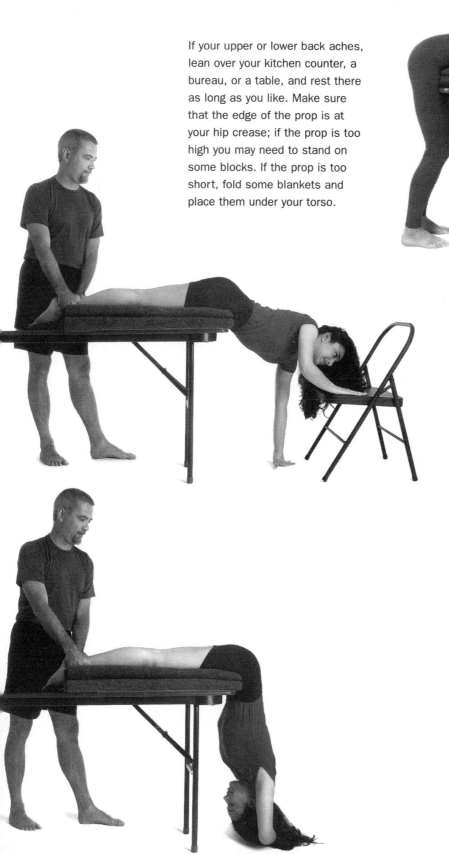

If your upper or lower back aches, lean over your kitchen counter, a bureau, or a table, and rest there as long as you like. Make sure that the edge of the prop is at your hip crease; if the prop is too high you may need to stand on some blocks. If the prop is too short, fold some blankets and place them under your torso.

Another cool trick to relieve back pain is to hang off the kitchen counter. Have a chair handy to help you get into and out of the position. Have a friend help you slide your hip crease to the edge and have your torso hang. Your friend should hold your legs so you don't completely slide off. If you are using a table or bureau that is shorter than the distance from your hip crease to the crown of your head, fold some blankets and place them on the table. Use a yoga mat under the blankets and on top of the blankets to prevent slipping.

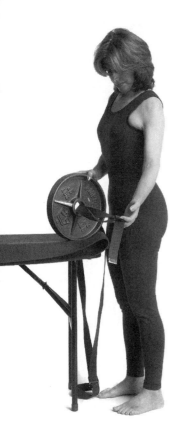

HAMSTRINGS AND SCIATICA

In this pose the quadriceps and femur bones are grounded, which allows the blood to circulate more freely in the hamstring. The increased circulation promotes healing of hamstring injuries and sciatica problems. This trick has helped me heal my own torn hamstring, and it has helped many students eliminate their sciatica pain after just a few practice sessions.

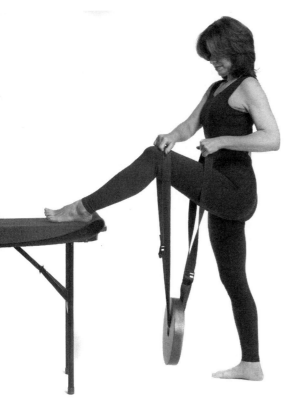

- Combine two yoga straps.

- Hold the two sides of the elongated strap together and pull through the center of the weight so that it will be at the midpoint of the straps.

- Stand facing a table or counter that is approximately the height of your hips. You should be a leg's distance from the table. Place a chair to one side of you. To help with balance, hold a chair the first few times you try this.

- Stand in Samasthithi. Shift your weight to the noninjured leg. Lift the injured leg and place your leg through the straps and place your heel directly in front of you on the table.

- Adjust the straps so that one strap is at the hip crease and the other is about two inches above the knee. The weight will hang in the center of your leg.

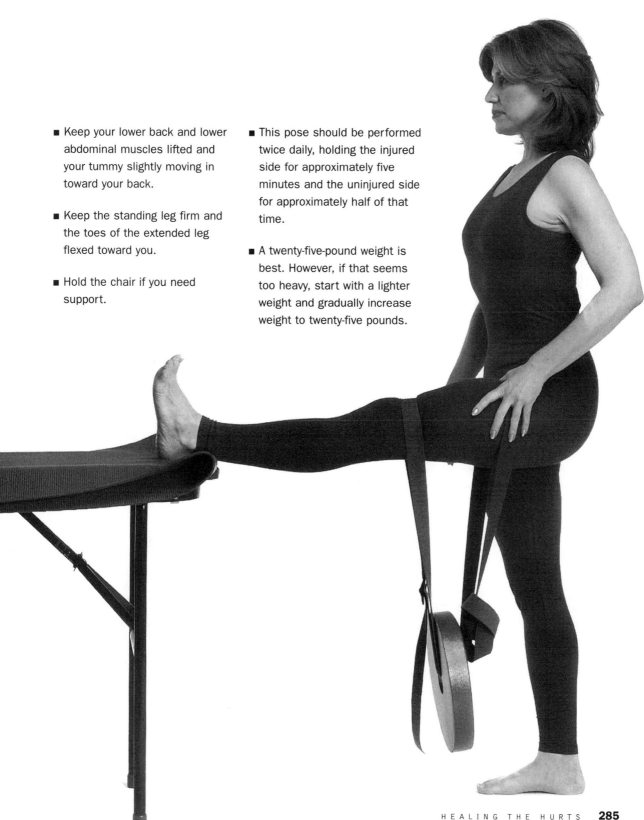

- Keep your lower back and lower abdominal muscles lifted and your tummy slightly moving in toward your back.

- Keep the standing leg firm and the toes of the extended leg flexed toward you.

- Hold the chair if you need support.

- This pose should be performed twice daily, holding the injured side for approximately five minutes and the uninjured side for approximately half of that time.

- A twenty-five-pound weight is best. However, if that seems too heavy, start with a lighter weight and gradually increase weight to twenty-five pounds.

About Our Models

All of our models practice yoga, some have for many, many years, some for much shorter periods of time. I am grateful to them for helping to produce such a beautiful book. It was great fun to work with all of you!

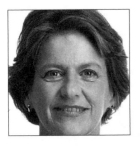

Nancy Crum Stechert came to yoga twenty-five years ago to stretch out after running marathons. The yoga stuck; the marathons went by the wayside. Nancy now lives in western Colorado where she teaches yoga and grows apples and cherries with her husband, Bob, and her two children, Jonathon and Annie. Nancy is Miriam's teacher.

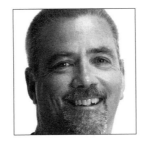

Terry Peterson has worked as a research scientist, forester, waiter, and garbageman. He thinks he has finally found the right job for him: teaching Iyengar-style yoga in Portland, Oregon. You can visit him at www.yogaterry.com.

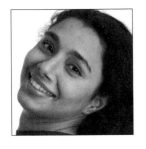

Having grown up in Bombay, **Nuvana Zarthoshtimanesh** started studying yoga as a young child. She recently moved to Portland, Oregon, with her new husband, Hormuzd Khosravi, where she studies and teaches Iyengar yoga.

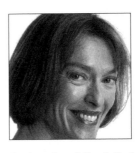

As founder of the **Julie Lawrence** Yoga Center in Portland, Oregon, Julie is busy teaching hundreds of yoga students each week—including most of the models in this book.

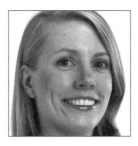

Maya Wells is a physical therapist who specializes in orthopedics and women's health. She used to be a modern/ballet dancer, many moons ago. Maya lives in Seattle with her husband, Herb, who is an inspiring third-grade teacher; their cat, Max; and their five-year-old goldfish, Wanda.

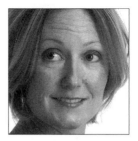

When not shopping at Nordstrom's, **Lynne McCandless** can be found practicing yoga, scuba diving, remodeling old homes, or cooking up a gourmet meal for friends with her husband, Aaron.

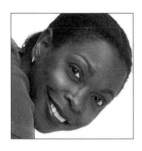

Mural Nishikawa started yoga to help ease her back pain. With a new baby and a demanding career as an internal medicine physician, Mural says yoga keeps her balanced, centered, and awake during the day.

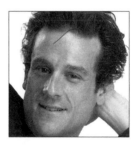

Jimmy Cohen devotes half of his professional time to developing real estate and the other half to helping troubled teens overcome their drug and alcohol addictions. In his spare time, Jimmy runs, bikes, lifts weights, and stretches out in Miriam's yoga classes in the Berkshire Hills of Massachusetts.

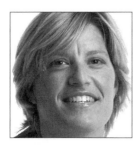

In addition to being a longtime student of Julie's, **Susan Hare** is a shiatsu massage therapist and a Zen practitioner.

Resources

To find a qualified teacher in your area, contact the Iyengar Yoga National Association of the United States at www.iynaus.org.

To learn more about healing illness and injury through yoga, refer to the book *Yoga: The Holistic Path to Health,* B.K.S. Iyengar, DK Books, 2001.

If you have any questions or comments, or want to learn more cool yoga tricks, contact Miriam Austin through her Web site: www.coolyogatricks.com.

To purchase yoga props, contact Miriam at her Web site or you can call her at 888-772-9642 (YOGA). One third of all profits from the sale of yoga props is used to provide food, medical care, and education to our brothers and sisters who are in the greatest need.

Index

About the Author

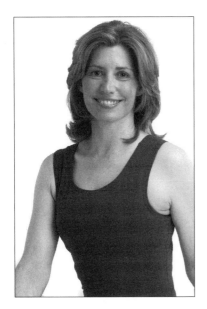

MIRIAM AUSTIN started studying yoga in 1985 as a way to de-stress from her successful yet high-pressure career in the investment business. Meditation was a natural extension of her yoga practice. Miriam now teaches yoga and meditation and writes books on these topics. She is also a fund-raiser for a not-for-profit organization that provides food, medical care, education, and spiritual direction for people in need throughout the world.